VDU Terminal Sickness

DEDICATED TO

my daughter, Linda Cheryl, without whose continuing support, encouragement and discussions the book would not have been written.

VDU Terminal Sickness

Computer health risks
and how to protect yourself

Peggy Bentham

GREEN
PRINT

First published in 1991 by
Green Print
an imprint of the Merlin Press
10 Malden Road, London NW5 3HR

ISBN 1 85425 043 4

Phototypeset by Computerset Ltd., Harmondsworth, Middlesex.

Printed in England by Biddles Ltd., Guildford, Surrey, on recycled paper.

Contents

ACKNOWLEDGEMENTS

I would like to acknowledge and express my thanks to all those who generously gave of their time for discussions, assistance and encouragement:

Jon Carpenter my publisher, Dr. Alan Michette, King's College, London, and Dr. Richard Lawson who raised some interesting questions and suggestions. Dr Leslie Hawkins, Robens Institute, Surrey University; Dr David Locke, United Kingdom Atomic Energy Association; Jack Shelmerdine, Radiological Protection Service, Manchester University; Prof. W.R. Lee, Professor of Occupational Health, Manchester University; Roger Blackwell, National Radiological Protection Board; John Phillips; Brian Pearce and Leslie Plant, Aston University, Birmingham; Geoffrey Bates, Fife Trading Standards Office; Tim Wells, National Computing Centre; Nicholas Winterton M.P.; George Teeling-Smith, Office of Health Economics, London; Nora King and Vi Gillman, National Back Pain Association, London; Dr. A.C. Mandal, Finsen Institute, Copenhagen; Dr. Rob L. Hendry, Kenmore Medical Centre, Wilmslow, Cheshire; Albert Hartley, Jo Rosenfeld and Chris Comer at Wilmslow Library, who persistently sought and acquired copies of several thousand scientific papers, journals and books from around the world; The staff at Manchester Reference library; Alex Lothian and David Smith from Open Systems Technology Europe Ltd; Steen Christensen of Incotel, London; Bob Norris of the National Union of Journalists; Marcus Bezzi of Stephens Innocent, London; Ann Inman and Kim Jones of Claremont Business Environments (Europe) Ltd., Warrington, Cheshire; Pete Worrall and Carl Munch from Broadstock Office Suppliers of Macclesfield; and Julian Hargreaves of Midas Office Designs of Marple, who each allowed me to test scores of different chairs and workstation formations and lighting from dozens of different manufacturers and for putting me in touch with others whose equipment they did not sell; Dr Scott Middleton and Dr Gowan Robinson of the British Chiropractic Association; Terry Mottershead of Granada Television; Marinus Kuik Snr., Marinus Kuik Jnr., Keith Dyson and Robert J. McCunney, The University Hospital, Boston, Massachusetts; Ken Ashton; the twins, Pamela and Patricia Dyson; Keith Dyson; Mark, Lisa and John Bentham.

I am also grateful to thousands of technologists, scientists, medical specialists, epidemiologists and reviewers, not named but who have conducted detailed research and produced so many diverse learned papers on the relevant aspects of the problems. The fact that so many excellent papers are not quoted in the book does not indicate that they are less relevant or valuable in any way than the ones that have been quoted, but simply there is now such a vast amount of evidence demonstrating various ill effects of VDUs that it would be impossible to quote from all the sources without extending the book into several weighty volumes.

To the following who granted permission to quote from their copyright of published work:

Elsevier Science Publishers, *Work With Display Units 86* (1987), edited by B Knave, and P.G. Widebäck.
Little, Brown & Co. Inc., Boston, Massachusetts, *Handbook of Occupational Medicine*, edited by Robert J McCunney.
BBC Television, to quote from the Panorama programme 'Electric City: A Shock In Store', presented by Tom Mangold, 21 March 1988.
Daniel Walker of N.C. Press Ltd., Toronto to quote from *Terminal Shock, The Health Hazards of Video Display Terminals*, Bob De Matteo, 1986.
Jack Simpson and the press office at the United Kingdom Atomic Energy Association, to quote from *Radiation Around Us*, and *The Effect and Control of Radiation*, 1988 and 1990.
John Wiley & Sons Ltd., *Health Hazards of VDUs?*, edited by Brian Pearce, 1984.

Introduction

The whole thing may end up like Three Mile Island. We won't know the extent of the damage for another ten to twenty years.

Unless VDU related health risks are resolved, and until new safety measures and working practices are introduced, the wonders of the new hi-tech age could result in the most unhealthy population in world history.

Millions of computer operators suffer from an assortment of health problems which occur after they start working with video display units (VDUs). Some of these problems occur within a few weeks or months of beginning to use the VDU, others develop over two or more years. Many of them are not serious in the long-term whilst others cause irreversible damage to the body. Some are classed as industrial injuries and qualify for disability pensions from the Department of Health and Social Security. Others could result in the premature loss of life itself!

Research figures reveal that over 90% of VDU operators suffer from one or more of the VDU-related health problems. They don't know exactly what is responsible for their deteriorating health. But they do know that something connected with working at the VDU is causing them to suffer health problems because, when they are away from their VDU for the weekend or a holiday, symptoms lessen and often disappear completely, only to recur once they go back to work.

It is estimated that within the next five years, over 70% of the working population in developed countries will use VDUs in the course of their work. Additionally, practically all schoolchildren today have been introduced to VDUs in the classroom, while ever-growing numbers have their own computers in the home.

Unless these health risks are resolved and until new safety measures and working practices are introduced, the wonders of the new hi-tech age could result in the most unhealthy population in world history.

Perhaps the general feeling is best summed up by a Newspaper Guild official who said,

The whole thing may end up like Three Mile Island. We won't know the extent of the damage for another ten or twenty years.

Yet, even now, there has been enough responsible scientific research conducted to show the way to reducing or avoiding most of these health risks.

Unfortunately, most reports produced by the specialists about their investigations and findings are not readily available to the general public. Nor are they easily understood by the layperson because of the scientific and technological jargon used.

This book interprets the available knowledge in jargon-free easily-understood terms, so that anyone working with VDUs and those members of management who are responsible for their purchase and installation can begin to understand why the health risks occur and then take positive steps to eliminate or avoid them.

1

Much of the research originates from many different countries. For that reason, and because the book will be available internationally, I should like to draw the reader's attention to the fact that the abbreviation VDU (video display unit) is the identifying description in Britain and several other countries for the computer screen. In those countries the term VDU terminal means the VDU along with the facilities in and around the place where the VDU is used (the work-station). In other countries, such as the USA, the computer screen itself is commonly known as a VDT (video display terminal), and the working environment as the VDT terminal or VDT work-station.

Because the book is intended to be practical rather than academic, detailed references have been kept to the end of the book, where they list the sources used so that readers interested in greater detail may consult the original research papers and articles.

PART ONE

The VDU

CHAPTER ONE
Progress brings new problems

Computers can seriously damage your health. Like cigarettes and alcohol, the fact that we might enjoy them is no guarantee that they are good for us. Particularly in excess.

During the past twenty-five years, most of us have been delighted to take advantage of some type of hi-tech electronic gadgetry; televisions, washing machines, dishwashers, food-mixers, microwave ovens, hair-dryers, calculators, fascinating toys for children, and so on. We introduced them into the home and the workplace with no thought of special facilities for them or of taking any precautions for our health against them – and none of us has appeared to suffer any ill-effects from our coveted, entertaining and labour-saving hi-tech acquisitions.

According to the 1990 report on a research study conducted by the Massachusetts Institute of Technology and the American National Institute of Standards and Technology, possible health risks from low level electromagnetic radiation emitted by many household products should be examined in much greater detail. There is not enough evidence to dismiss potential health risks from weak electromagnetic fields found around many domestic appliances, power lines and computers.

Everything connected to the electricity supply emits one or more types of electromagnetic radiation into the surrounding atmosphere. Some of these can interfere with other equipment, and possibly our health. A report by the American Environmental Protection Agency, published in *Nature* in June 1990, says of this type of electromagnetic pollution that 'studies of leukaemia, lymphoma and brain cancer in children exposed to magnetic fields from residential 60Hz electrical power-distribution systems, supported by similar findings in adults . . . show a consistent pattern of response'.

Few of us suspect that these invisible electromagnetic waves (sometimes referred to as electronic pollution or electronic smog) surround us in our homes and general environment.

There are cases where a security guard's walkie-talkie has caused a firm's computer to crash. The waves emanating from hair dryers and other domestic equipment frequently cause televisions, telephones and radios to crackle. A computer in one room can interfere with sensitive hospital equipment in an adjoining room. Electromagnetic waves at ground level have even been recorded to interfere with electronic controls in aircraft.

If you walk around your office or home with one of the new cordless telephones switched on, you will be able to hear crackles as you pass or stand in potentially dangerous areas where there is a build-up of electromagnetic radiation.

In January 1992, new European legislation will come into effect which will outlaw electrical appliances whose electromagnetic waves interfere with other electrical equipment in the vicinity. From that date it will be a legal requirement that new products are tested for compatibility and immunity from interference.

Unfortunately, there are millions of pieces of equipment already on the market which really ought to be checked, but since there are so very few sites in Britain that are equipped to test them, it seems likely that existing equipment will remain hazardous.

Domestic appliances are extremely simple in comparison to most computers and their VDUs. Nonetheless, we do not continually sit two or three feet away from them – for up to eight hours per day, five days each week, year in and year out!

A new environment is essential for VDUs

There are some ill-informed and unsuspecting people – even managements – who seem to regard the VDU as a combination of a glass typewriter and a sophisticated calculator.

The personal computer and its VDU is not a new sophisticated hi-tech gadget which we can simply place on the desk in the existing office or home environment and plug into the electricity supply.

Pre-existing work methods, office design, lighting, furnishings and the quality of the surrounding air are not only quite unsuitable for working with VDUs, they can also contribute to new health problems.

Ignorance of this has been responsible for some VDU operators being exposed to unnecessary suffering. Frequently computer salesmen, and even accountancy staff acting in an advisory capacity, deliberately neglect to tell buyers that existing surroundings and working practices are unlikely to be suitable for working with the VDU. Their commissions on sales might be lost if the client realised that the cost of the computer, VDU and printer were only a small part of the necessary financial outlay required – both to take advantage of the wonders of the computer age and to protect the operator's health and well-being. Some irresponsible firms of accountants advise clients to buy new equipment but then make no provision in their clients' figures for these additional costs!

Equally, there are a number of penny-pinching employers and schools who often know better, but whose aim is to take advantage of the new computer technology with the minimum financial outlay. They look to buy the cheapest equipment which they put on an existing desk or table space, and they then expect a secretary or typist to fathom the whole lot out from voluminous, weighty and often incomprehensible manuals, without changing the working environment.

Transferable keyboard skills

No one should expect secretarial or typewriter keyboard skills to be transferable to the task of operating a computer without a considerable amount of retraining. It is irrelevant that both the typewriter and computer are used for communication purposes and that each has a keyboard.

The driving skills and experience of the driver and footman of the horse-drawn carriage became irrelevant when the motor car was introduced. Both modes of transport were concerned with travel, horsepower and wheels, but skills of that bygone era were not readily transferable to safely driving and maintaining the motor car. Similarly past typewriter keyboard experience is inadequate and inappropriate for many of the skills required by the VDU operator.

VDUs can seriously damage your health

Certainly the working tasks which the computer performs appear to be almost miraculous. From this point of view, no one who has mastered the art of operating a computer in the course of their work would really like to go back to working without one. And I include myself. But then, like cigarettes and alcohol, the fact that we might enjoy them is no guarantee that they are good for us. Particularly in excess.

Who is at risk?

It has been estimated that by the turn of the century at least two out of every three people who work will use a VDU for some part of their work. Already they appear on the desks of most doctors in their surgeries, they have become common in schools, in every branch of management, design studios, and virtually every professional and occupational group. Everyone who uses a VDU is exposed to risk.

Some groups of people are more susceptible to harmful effects in the VDU workplace than others. Some operators will suffer absolutely no adverse health effects whatsoever. By no means will everybody who works with a VDU suffer from any one particular health problem.

Few of us fit the specification used in tests of 'the average person' for whom most equipment is designed. Few of us can be constantly classed as the perfect, healthy, average-sized human being. From the outset most of us have different physical strengths, defects and weaknesses, shapes and sizes. And these need to be catered for.

Some people suffering from recognised pre-existing medical conditions are warned that they should *never* use a VDU. They include:

1 Anyone who is fitted with a pace-maker.
2 Those who do, or might, suffer from photosensitive epilepsy.
3 Women who are pregnant, or those who are hoping to become pregnant in the near future.

If working with the VDU was completely harmless, the above three groups of people would be able to be exposed like the rest of us.

Study of available evidence and personal knowledge leads me to believe that it is the most efficient operators who are likely to suffer most.

Men and passive users

Research clearly demonstrates that people, particularly men, who do not work at the VDU, but who spend considerable amounts of time in the office environment where VDUs are in use, could be subjected to an assortment of detrimental effects relating to their health in general and to their virility and fertility in particular. Men are more at risk than women, because the male genitals are not so well-protected by the outer body as are those of females.[13-16,23-25] Knowledge of this possibility alone usually helps to concentrate senior managements' attention to the VDU health problems – giving new meaning to the executive brief![22]

Children, parents and teachers

Many parents have bought personal computers for home use. At the beginning of 1988 a survey revealed that 25% of teenage boys and 11% of teenage girls had their own. Often these home VDUs and those in schools are used in circumstances which are far from ideal.

Of particular interest and importance to those responsible for children using computers is the, as yet, unanswered question of whether the growing bodies of children are more likely to suffer ill-effects than adults. Also, whether the current safety standards laid down offer sufficient protection for children. In relation to children, two developments give cause for concern. The first is that, though extremely rare, the use of computers could trigger off photosensitive epilepsy. This is most likely to occur in children between the ages of 10 and 14. Most first attacks occur before the age of 20.

Secondly, in May 1988 specialists in paediatrics and radiology (from the Great Ormond Street children's hospital) reported that the level of medical X-rays previously considered safe for children is now in serious doubt. They claim that 'their life expectancy is long, allowing more time for radiation-induced cancers to appear. Their tissues show increased radiosensitivity'. Dr Christine Hall, consultant paediatric radiologist and Dr Richard Dawood, senior registrar at Great Ormond Street, the consultants concerned, have proposed alternatives to any exposure to X-rays for children for medical purposes. These specialists feel that ultrasound and magnetic resonance imaging should be used instead of X-rays for performing medical examinations on children.[1] Herein lies an insight into just one of the current anxieties, since VDUs undeniably emit measurable quantities of X-rays. Some VDUs have been taken off the market because they were found to exceed the officially recommended safety levels for X-rays.[2-4]

What causes the problems?

One survey demonstrates that only 5% to 10% of VDU workers operate under ideal healthy conditions. The main health problems stem from the facts that:

1 VDUs emit *eight* different categories of electromagnetic radiation in measurable quantities. The VDU operator is working in a pulsating electromagnetic field and is exposed to varying amounts of static electricity.[3,5]
2 Established working practices, which have been suitable for secretarial and managerial office work, can be extremely harmful to operators. New working practices are absolutely necessary.[6,7,11]
3 The office layout, lighting, furniture and sundry equipment and tools need to be specially designed and installed to protect the operator's health.[6-10,12]
4 The electricity supply must be a constant and clean line with no peaks, surges and troughs. Our mains electricity supply does not meet this required standard.
5 Hi-tech equipment, furnishings and recommended acceptable safe levels of radiation exposure are designed for the perfectly healthy average human being. Not all operators conform to this standard all of the time – if at all.
6 The operator must be able to control the purity and temperature of the air in which he or she is working. They must be able to control atmospheric changes attributable to the various aspects of the sick building syndrome brought about from over-zealous energy conservation measures and natural variable atmospheric factors like changing weather conditions.[7]
7 Today, inadequate repair services are frequently masquerading as servicing facilities. Additionally, servicing personnel are often not equipped to carry out the requisite tests for fluctuating power supply, or to perform adequate radiation tests on the equipment.

Later chapters examine and analyse all of these problems in detail and show how steps can be taken to eliminate or avoid most of them.

How common are the health risks?

Assorted health problems directly related to using a VDU became so repetitive on an international scale that responsible major companies, assorted bureaucratic bodies, technologists, doctors, multidisciplinary medical specialists and other groups of scientists started to do controlled research projects searching for the explanations for these new health risks. Scientists from the USA, Canada, Australia, Japan, Sweden and Britain have been particularly active in this field.

Groups of scientists from around the world have organised meetings to compare progress in their particular specialised areas of study. At one such ergonomics conference held in Manchester in 1983, the Swedish delegates proposed that a major world conference be organised to address the VDU health risks and should be attended by world leaders in all of the disciplinary specialisations who were involved in finding solutions.

Professor Etienne Grandjean, from Zurich, a pioneer in the field of ergonomics, was consulted and asked to be the international honorary co-ordinator of the first world conference. As a result of this, the first international scientific conference took place in Stockholm in May 1986, when 1,200 delegates from 35 countries gathered together to report on their progress and reveal their findings.

Contradictory voices

During the course of all scientific research it is common for different opinions and conclusions to be reached by different groups of experts, even within each specialisation itself. There are often prolonged periods of time when scientists criticise and disagree with their colleagues' working methods and conclusions. Over the very many years it takes for these investigations and field research to be completed, overwhelming evidence continues to be presented in reports – written in scientific, technical and technological terms – which demonstrate that the health problems are serious and worsening. The available knowledge could begin to be put to good use to ease or avoid some of the health problems. But it is not. The reports have a very limited specialist circulation and they neither reach nor are understood by those who most need to know.

After many of the health problems are recognised and accepted – and whilst all this extensive and serious research into those problems is taking place – there are still some manufacturers, employers, doctors and regulatory bodies who attempt to use their authority to try to persuade suffering VDU operators that there is no evidence to suggest that working with a VDU could be responsible for any detrimental effects to their health. With a carefully studied and rehearsed play on ambiguous terminology they claim that either the operators are imagining their health problems or that these are attributable to some other cause. At the same time, authoritative voices denounce the increasing international flow of news-paper and magazine features on this subject as scare stories.

One common put-off line is that operators' problems might stem from a deep-rooted psychological distrust and dislike of having to learn to use computers. Yet I know quite definitely that fresh flowers die alongside my own VDU within a few hours of being placed there, whilst identical flowers cut at the same time and placed in an adjoining computer-less room live more than ten times longer. All the other factors relating to these flowers are identical. And presumably we can all accept that flowers do not have psychological problems about being placed close to computers or computer screens.

Déjà vu

Official statements denying that a serious health risk exists, combined with the continually deteriorating collective health of workers, is not without precedent. Since the days when the ancient Greeks decreed that 'working is bad for the health', industrial progress has been littered with occupational health problems causing physical suffering and death.

Numerous workers are repeatedly exposed to dangerous situations and suffer deteriorating health problems. Some die whilst bureaucratic health and safety bodies and industry drag their feet and make utterances which, ambiguously to the layperson, convey the meaning that they are satisfied that no health problem exists.

Comparatively recently we remember the tragic saga of asbestos and its related health problems. Despite repeated international complaints and a growing death toll of workers, evidence about the risk to millions of workers was officially deliberately suppressed, even although medical researchers linked asbestos exposure to severe scarring of the lung tissue as long ago as 1920 and to lung cancer in 1935. By the 1970s, more than eleven million workers had been unnecessarily and irresponsibly exposed to asbestos since the end of the Second World War. It is anticipated that in the case of asbestos compensation to sufferers and relatives of the deceased will far exceed $2 billion.[20]

Equally our trust in the safety of medical practices and products has been misplaced as in the cases of Distillers' Thalidomide, with appalling suffering to its 402 victims costing £32.5 million in compensation, and many others such as Eli Lilly's Opren and ICI's Eraldin.

VDU operators' legal battles

Over the past few years, in Australia and the USA there have been innumerable cases of VDU operators taking legal proceedings against employers and computer manufacturers, seeking recompense in the courts for damage which they have suffered to their health as a direct result of their work at the screen. Most of the cases have been successful, resulting in substantial financial damages being awarded to the operators. A few cases have been unsuccessful. The great majority of claims for compensation have been settled out of court.

In Britain, the first such case was brought in May 1989 by Mrs Pauline Burnard, of Nottingham. She suffered so badly from tenosynovitis (a repetitive strain injury) that she was compelled to retire from work at the age of 30.[26] Pauline's case was supported and presented by the Banking Insurance and Finance union. She was awarded £45,000 damages in the High Court against her employer, Midland Bank.

Another case was heard in the Lewes Crown Court, Sussex, in March 1990. £107,500 damages were awarded to three women computer workers who sued their employers, the Inland Revenue office in Durrington, West Sussex.

At the *Financial Times* some journalists suffering from the painful arm, hand and wrist conditions have been off work for three years on fully salary. Backed by the NUJ, several of these journalists have served writs against the newspaper, seeking compensation.

By mid-July 1991, the FT prepared to pay off RSI victims with substantial payments of around £140-150,000. Managing editor David Walker acknowledged: 'There is a need to face up to the fact that, for some people, it may be the case that they may not be able to work again as journalists on the FT.'

Within a few days, Reuters similarly made a settlement of £200,000 for RSI damages to another journalist who brought a law suit against them.

Bob Norris (the legal eagle of the British National Union of Journalists) has been inundated with calls for help from afflicted journalists at their VDU screens. On their behalf, the numbers of individual cases against famous newspapers now progressing through the legal system are well into the hundreds and rising. The NUJ scribes are in the capable hands of Marcus Bezzi (now based at the firm of Stephens Innocent in London), a well-known Australian lawyer with a vast amount of successful litigation in this specialised field.

Marcus Bezzi told me: 'The cases which we are representing now will start to be heard in the British courts during 1991 and 1992. Of course, many employers are offering financial settlements out of court.'

I asked if he was able to quantify the problems. He replied:

'It is impossible to put an average figure on the compensation amounts, because that would be pro rata to the degree of injury and the rate of earnings. Many of the journalists I am representing earn considerably more than the cases that have been publicised, therefore the compensation in each case would be expected to be considerably higher.'

Taking the RSI injury rate in isolation, it appears that amongst newspaper staff a very conservative estimate would be that 10% are seriously afflicted by repetitive strain injuries. Translated on a global scale with over 82 million VDU users, this could lead to compensation claims of over £1 billion from this category of complaints alone.

Trying to get compensation through the courts has been a daunting, time-consuming, complex and expensive task in the past. Now it is less so since most trade unions are taking on cases for their members and legal aid is available in Britain to many others who have a viable case and who otherwise could not afford to take legal action.

Additionally, maybe the insurance industry will become a watch-dog over client companies' health and safety procedures, since an amendment to the Companies Bill in 1989 now makes them liable for compensation to workers, even if the company has gone into liquidation – and even if symptoms do not appear until years after the VDU operator's employment ceased,[21] which is not uncommon with radiation-linked health problems.

Hopefully, it will be a strong deterrent to cavalier employers and manufacturers alike, to learn of the ever-increasing numbers of successful legal cases and of the often vast sums of money awarded in compensation by the courts to VDU operators who have suffered from some of these health problems and from a deterioration to the quality of life, and of their far-reaching liability for years ahead.

Nonetheless, even when litigation is successful, it is unlikely that there can ever be adequate compensation for prolonged suffering which reduces the quality of life, or for irreversible deterioration in health that sometimes leads even to the loss of life itself.

Unfortunately, so far as VDUs are concerned, it would appear that we are unlikely to know the true extent of the damage for another ten or even twenty years because (a) radiation damage is cumulative and additive, and even if people cease to be exposed to the risks it can take several years before some of the problems develop fully and become obvious, (as was the case in those exposed to asbestos); and (b) because of the number of years it takes for bureaucratically acceptable epidemiological tests to be finalised.

Health and safety

No one should allow the quality of their health and their life to deteriorate by harmful working conditions. If you suspect that you are suffering from a medical problem related to your work you should:

1 Consult your own doctor.
2 Report the problem to your employer.
3 Report the problem to the Health and Safety Executive. Under the Diseases and Dangerous Occurrences Regulations 1985 (RIDDOR), accidents and illness at work must be reported – it's the law.
4 If you are a member of a trade union, report it to them.
5 Take preventative action – if possible. This book will help you to do that.
6 If you or your employer is unwilling or unable to take the requisite preventative action, the only sensible thing to do is to immediately stop doing the work – or working in the environment which causes the problem.[17-19]

The family doctor

Doctors and specialists should be familiar with the majority of the medical complaints VDU operators suffer from. They are accustomed to recognising and treating most of them. Nonetheless it augurs well to remember that their professional responsibility is to treat the symptoms but not to conduct research into just how, where or why the symptoms arose. However, if you feel that your deteriorating health is attributable to your work, you should tell your doctor this – and give your reasons for suspecting that this is so.

Relating health problems to working with VDUs is a fairly recent idea. Whilst most doctors now understand the connections and are sympathetic, there is still a small body of doctors who would not acknowledge that the problems are caused by the computer working environment. Numerous operators have come to me for help, after they have received neither help nor understanding from their own doctor. From them I have learned that, regrettably, there are still some doctors who quote the official line which is that 'from the information available, VDUs do not cause health problems'. Another common response is that 'if you are sure that the problem is VDU-related – stop working on a VDU'. Which is, of course, exactly what growing numbers of operators are doing.

Unfortunately there are still not enough family doctors who are either trained or experienced in industrial hygiene or medicine (the medical specialisation for detecting and treating the ever increasing range of work-related illnesses). If your doctor has not got this experience then you should be advised to consult one who has.

Staff and skill shortages

A common complaint amongst employers is that there is a 33% annual turnover in VDU staff. Those companies who do have a high level of VDU operators leaving are usually guilty of providing inferior or faulty equipment, a poor working environment and of having unrealistic expectations of human ability and endurance. In short, most of these employers suffer from the unrealistic, uninformed, penny-pinching 'glass typewriter' misconception – which this book will examine in detail as it progresses.

Internationally, new hi-tech recruitment agencies have opened. The demand for their services, and consequently the agencies' profits, are growing fast. They are specialising in contracting out temporary hi-tech operators to fill the vacancies and to attempt to eliminate the staff shortages. It is interesting to scan the recruitment columns placed by these agencies in newspapers. In the course of 1990 the salary levels offered to attract the requisite staff tripled.

Meanwhile, desperate and unprecedented new initiatives were launched in March 1990 in a campaign by the UK computer industry, the Women into Information Technology Committee (which was backed by the Department of Trade and Industry), and BBC TV. These initiatives are to promote careers in technology to schoolgirls and those returning to work after having families. As a precedent to the launch, schools throughout the country were asked to encourage their pupils to compete in computer competitions. Tempting prizes were won.

CHAPTER TWO
Some VDUs are potential killers

Twenty-five percent of computers tested failed basic safety tests. Considering that research figures reveal sales in excess of 82 million VDUs that means that, in 1991, there could be over twenty million faulty VDUs being used by completely unsuspecting operators.

There is no legal requirement in Britain for computers and their VDUs to be tested for safety before they are sold to the public. Richard Smith and his team of computer testing consultants in Dunfermline claim that tens of thousands of computers and VDUs currently in use could be potentially lethal because of design and manufacturing faults.

The Scottish consultancy is part of an international network of hi-tech consultancy companies who operate together under the name of Open Systems Technology (Europe) Ltd. Working to government guidelines OST (and other similar groups) test computers and VDUs, principally to determine whether different manufacturers' models will be able to communicate with each other in accordance with open system information (OSI) standards.

Alex Lothian, the chairman of OST, told me that there are thousands of faulty and dangerous computers and VDUs in use in Britain alone, the products of at least a score of different manufacturers. He would like to see a change in the law to make it compulsory for all manufacturers to have their equipment tested to ensure that all components and systems conform to safety standards before the computers are allowed to be sold to the consumer, and to compel manufacturers to have all existing equipment in use inspected – and modified where necessary – to meet these standards.

In May 1990, whilst Richard Smith and his team were diligently performing standard compatibility tests on various types of computers and VDUs, they performed additional tests for user safety, to ensure that computer operators and service engineers will not get an electric shock, and to check that the equipment won't burst into flames and burn the building down. On this occasion, personal computers from two manufacturers seriously failed to comply with low voltage safety regulations made under the 1989 Consumer Protection Act. If there is a mains power surge, the insulation on these VDUs would break down. The operator and service engineers would be exposed to severe electric shock. Smith says: 'These VDUs are potential killers.'

Considerable numbers of these dangerous units had already been sold and were being used by unsuspecting operators.

Within days of the reports being issued the two manufacturers in question assured OST that all the dangerous equipment which had been sold was either being recalled or engineers were being sent out to customers' premises to make the equipment safe. Additionally assurances were given that their overseas manufacturing bases would modify future models to comply with British safety regulations.

Unsafe equipment is commonplace

Alex Lothian explained that it is not uncommon for computer equipment to breach British Standards Institution safety tests – sometimes quite seriously. Too many manufacturers put profitability before safety.

In cases where public safety does become a concern, OST compiles detailed reports and copies are sent – confidentially – to the manufacturer concerned and to assorted regulatory agencies, including the consumer safety units of the Department of Trade and Industry. Because the information is confidential it is not possible to publish lists of offending manufacturers. Normally manufacturers of faulty equipment take immediate steps to ensure that modifications are made.

Geoff Bates, a senior inspector at Fife trading standards department in Scotland, confirms that there is no requirement for electrical equipment to be tested for safety before being put on to the market. However, he says,

Manufacturers and distributors who do knowingly breach the safety regulations are committing a criminal offence. The 1989 Consumer Protection Act was intended to bring British regulations into line with European safety standards which demand that electrical equipment must be adequately earthed and insulated. And, that proper instructions are provided for safe operation of electrical equipment.

What you can do to protect yourself

Asked for advice on what consumers should do if they suspect that all is not as it should be with their computer equipment, Mr Bates advises:

1 Complain to your local trading standards department whose address can be found in the telephone directory, usually under the name of your county council. Tell them about the fault. They will need evidence of place and date of purchase and to know that the equipment has not been tampered with by an unqualified person.
2 If, when the local trading standards department has completed its own test, the equipment is found to be dangerous, they will serve suspension notices on that manufacturer which will enforce removal of those models from the market.
3 If personal injury has been suffered, managements or manufacturers can be sued for product liability under the Consumer Protection Act 1987. Legal action for personal injury may be taken by the local environmental health department if the defendant's staff numbers fifteen people or less; or, by the Health and Safety Executive for all larger companies and organisations.

OST say that 25% of the computers they have tested failed basic safety tests. Given worldwide sales in excess of 82 million VDUs, that means that, in 1991, there are over twenty million faulty VDUs in circulation being used by completely unsuspecting operators.

CHAPTER THREE
Where the problems come from

The VDU is not a typewriter with a glass screen. It is a radiation-emitting
device and its use requires entirely different environmental conditions and
working practices from a typewriter.

If we are simply concerned with operating the VDU it is not necessary to
understand its basic construction and internal workings. However, so that we
may understand how health problems arise from these VDU sources, it is helpful
to know a little about the construction of the VDU and its keyboard, and the way
they work, so that we can begin to understand how and why they can quite
seriously interfere with our health and wellbeing.

The computer system is made up of four separate pieces of equipment
connected with cables. They are:

1 The VDU, which looks like a small television and is in fact constructed in
   a similar way to a television.
2 The keyboard, which is similar to a typewriter keyboard in that the
   alphabetic letters are laid out in the same QWERTY order. But this
   keyboard has many more keys, because the computer can perform
   different and very many more functions than the typewriter. There is also
   a great difference in the angle and tilt of the keyboard.
3 At least one printer, usually situated fairly close to the VDU.
4 The computer (an electronics circuit pack) which might be situated on the
   desk underneath the VDU, as in the case of a small personal computer;
   or, if it is a large computer being used by several people, it might be
   situated in a different room or even a different building.

These four pieces of equipment are individually encased in their own metal,
plastic or fibreglass casing. The computer industry buzzword for any of these
pieces of equipment, singly or collectively, is 'hardware'.

The whole system comes to life when it is plugged into the electricity power
supply.

Recognisable sources of eyestrain, headaches and muscular problems

Before we begin to consider what is inside the VDU and how it works, we know
that we would not watch television in the same bright lighting conditions which
we would use for general work or for writing or reading. When we watch
television most of us either partly draw curtains or dim the room lighting so that
the image on the screen can be seen clearly. We would not watch a TV screen for
very long if furnishings or bright lights from the room were reflected on it, and

15

certainly not with sunlight shining on to it, or if the contrast on the screen was bad or if there was a glare or a flicker on the screen. If we did view under any of these adverse conditions, we certainly would not do so for several hours in the day, every day of the working week.

Immediately then, we know that normal room lighting is usually far too bright for pleasant – or safe – viewing of the VDU. Working under the wrong lighting conditions can cause varied eye problems and it can also be responsible for mild to severe headaches.

If the room lighting conditions are not perfect for viewing it is natural for us to try to compensate by inclining the head to one side – perhaps to cut out a reflection – or to move the body to a different angle so that the offending reflection is reduced or eliminated. If we remain in that odd position for any length of time, this can cause a variety of muscular problems in neck and back.

Earlier I mentioned the physical imperfections of the human VDU operator. A very common physical defect relates to our eyesight. Operators who wear spectacles which have been prescribed for reading or distance viewing will need to have their eyes re-tested for VDU work. Most people with imperfect vision will need new spectacles to be made for the exact working distance between their eyes and the VDU screen. The screen is at a distance and angle at which we are not accustomed to viewing and for which reading or general distance spectacles will not be suitable. Failure to be able to view the screen from a well supported seated position, without leaning the head or body forward, will result in eyestrain, headaches and muscular problems.

The screen must be placed on a tilt and swivel stand so that the operator can adjust its vertical and horizontal position to get the best viewing angle for their personal physical shape, eyesight and position. The screen must be quite separate from the keyboard so that both can be positioned at variable, both physically and visually comfortable distances for your eyes and fingers.

Inside the VDU

Like a television, the VDU is constructed around a cathode-ray tube, or CRT, which is basically a glass tube with a cathode (electron gun) at one end and a screen coated in phosphor at the other.

When a high electrical voltage reaches the cathode a stream of electrons is produced. This stream of electrons passes through a grid which modulates its intensity, then through two or three anodes which accelerate and focus the stream of electrons into a beam (rather like the light passing through a camera lens). The focused beam then passes through electrostatic or electromagnetic deflecting devices in or around the neck of the tube which, in turn, direct the electron beam to the required position on the screen.

The impact of the electron beam on the phosphor coating of the screen produces a bright spot of light visible to the viewer.

The visual quality of the words or pictures displayed on the screen is dependent upon the efficiency of the phosphor on the inside of the screen.

Two procedures produce the pictures, words and figures. First, a saw-tooth magnetic field is applied to the vertical deflector system. This field lowers the electron beam down the screen and then returns the beam to the upper limit of the screen, sixty times per second. This frequency governs the 'refresh rate' of the screen information. (Simply, that means the number of scan lines on the screen. In the USA, TV and VDU screens have 525 scan lines, whilst the UK and Europe use 625 lines). The vertical deflector system produces a pulsed extremely low frequency (ELF) field of the type that a leading American scientist claims has the propensity to damage brain tissues in humans.[27]

Second, a saw-tooth magnetic field 'flyback' moves the beam from the left to the right of the screen 15,000 to 20,000 times per second, producing a very low frequency (VLF) field of 15 to 20 kHz. This field is generated by the flyback transformer and is applied to the horizontal deflecting system.

These frequencies of electromagnetic radiation have been found to cause an assortment of detrimental health effects which are explained in detail in Part 3.

Residual gases, ions and several types of electromagnetic radiation are produced within the tube; these are also discussed fully in Part 3.

The VDU screen is sealed off to maintain a vacuum. It consists of two layers. The first is a metal layer with a high potential which accelerates the electrons in the final part of their trajectory. It also reflects light from the phosphor towards the operator and increases the brightness of the image. Another layer is made up of fluorescent screen material where the electron energy is converted to light.

The glass envelope of the VDU is conductive and has a permalloy layer, to shield the tube from electrostatic and magnetic fields. The permalloy shield is an alloy (a mixture of metals) of nickel and iron, often containing other elements such as copper, molybdenum and chromium. It is used to stop the electromagnetic radiation produced within the VDU by the deflection coils and the flyback transformer from entering the cathode-ray tube.

Hot work

All electrical and electronic equipment generates heat when it is switched on and working. The average electric typewriter generates about 35 watts. The average VDU generates about 400 watts. Most VDUs are equipped with an internal fan to provide air circulation and cooling within the terminal cabinet, which has ventilation grilles to allow air to flow freely into and out of the terminal.

The amount of heat generated by the VDU can raise the room temperature quite noticeably, at the same time lowering the humidity of the air. In those offices and schools where a number of VDUs are being used in the same room this can be one of the causes of assorted skin problems (including ageing effects), irritable and pink eyes, sore throats, respiratory problems and general discomfort.

If the VDU is allowed to overheat the efficiency of the electronic components is affected which can result in total breakdown of the equipment.

Radiation

The performance of the cooling fan can also alter the levels of radiation which are emitted from the VDU. Therefore you must never be tempted to put papers or books on top of the VDU casing (which often happens because of lack of desk space) because this would detrimentally interfere with the all-important air circulation and cooling system.

The multiplicity of health problems which can arise from radiation are so numerous that separate chapters are devoted to them – advising how to recognise most of the danger signs and how to avoid them.

What you can do

1 Be sure the screen stands on an adjustable tilt and swivel stand that allows you to move it both horizontally and vertically to suit your physical size and eyesight.
2 Don't use a VDU unless you can see the screen easily when you are sitting back in your chair without squinting, bending or twisting your body.
3 Ensure that the room and work-top lighting levels can be adjusted to suit you. Those operators whose lighting conditions have not been designed for working at the VDU should refer to Chapter 25.
4 Have you had your eyes tested to ensure that either your natural eyesight or your spectacles are correct for the exact, unusual and unaccustomed viewing distance between eyes and screen?
5 Ensure that both the screen and the keyboard are separate items of equipment so that each can separately be adjusted to an angle and position that are comfortable to your individual physical characteristics.
6 High quality, sharp, clearly defined letters and figures displayed on an absolutely flicker-free screen are absolutely vital to the VDU operator's well-being. If your screen does not meet all of these requirements your health could be at risk. Do not use the VDU. Call in a service engineer. And read Chapters 13, 14 and 15 for further guidance.
7 Equally, nobody should work on a screen if the lines of text appear to bend or fade away.
8 The operator must have the ability to adjust the contrast and brightness of the work displayed on the screen. If you are uncertain how to do this, refer to the checklist in Chapter 15.
9 Every inch of the screen must be absolutely evenly illuminated.

Health Note: failure to adhere to the above safety standards can cause a range of serious health risks.

CHAPTER FOUR
The printer

The noise from one daisywheel printer exceeds the health and safety level set by the British civil service union.

Several health problems can be attributed to placing the printer close to the operator. These include stress, tinnitus, deafness, headaches, nausea, smarting and itching eyes, nasal problems, damage to the cells of the airways of the lungs, bronchitis, sore throats, skin rashes, eczema, premature ageing, irritation and depression of the central nervous system, convulsions and loss of consciousness.

Ideally printers, like photocopiers, should be placed in a separate well-ventilated soundproof room where they cannot contribute to air pollution or increased noise levels.

If printers are put in the same room as operators they should be at least 3 to 4 metres away from any workers and ought to be provided with their own air extraction to take noxious fumes right out of the working atmosphere. Danish scientists say that laser printers could be emitting levels of toxic ozone ten times higher than the British safety standards.

Poisonous gases from laser printers

Whilst the depletion of ozone levels in the upper atmosphere causes concern, few realise that laser printers and photocopiers are emitting potentially harmful ozone into the air in offices. In Scandinavia a series of comprehensive tests has been carried out on laser printers and copiers and it has been established that the emissions of ozone, dust and, to a lesser extent, heat can create serious health problems. It is fairly well recognised that these noxious effects may be a significant threat to office workers.

Ozone is a toxic gas with a distinctive odour and is a normal, albeit minute, constituent of the earth's atmosphere. It is produced naturally from oxygen whenever ultraviolet radiation or high voltage electrical discharges occur. The high voltage applied in the printing and copying processes of laser printers and copiers creates ozone.

The concentration of ozone from a laser printer is between 0.1 and 1.2 ppm (parts per million). In the UK the Health and Safety Executive recommends a safety level of an exposure limit of 0.1 ppm averaged over an eight hour day, with no fifteen minutes peak greater than 0.3 ppm,[26] which should trigger a warning signal to you that with continued use the laser printer will progressively heat causing an increasingly higher emission of radiation and ozone.

There is more information about ozone and safety levels in Chapter 14.

Ozone extraction safety filters

Most laser printers have a built-in filter to extract the ozone from the exhaust fumes. However these filters are often inadequate and do not completely break down the ozone. Additionally, their effectiveness is reduced if they are not discarded and replaced frequently (every three to six months depending on use), or if they are subjected to an environment containing dust, tobacco smoke and other airborne pollutants.

Table 4.1 The effect of exposure to ozone on humans and animals

Concentration (ppm)	Time exposed	Health effects
0.008 to 0.02	instantly	threshold of smell
0.08	3 hours	increased mortality rate for mice from lung infection
0.1	short time	eye irritation for humans
0.1	short time	dryness in upper respiratory passages – irritation in nose and throat in humans
0.2	5 hrs a day over 3 weeks	structural damages to heart tissues in mice and rats
0.2 to 0.5	single 3 hour exposure, or two 3 hour exposures with 1 hour interval	negative effect on the optic nerve
0.2 to 0.25	30 minutes	red blood cells affected in humans, mice, rats and rabbits
0.28	30 minutes	distinct dryness of the throat and tickling in the nose
0.37	2 hours	increased resistance in the upper respiratory passages and diminished ventilation of the lungs
0.2 to 0.8	2 hours	several similar experiments reported a reduction in the function of the lungs, and irritation of the nose, eyes and throat
0.2 to 0.8	2 hours	5%-25% change in the function of the lungs
0.3 to 0.8	chronic exposure	an increased number of welding operators registered complaints of tightness in chest and irritation of the throat as well as severe headaches
1.5 to 2.0	2 hours	extreme chest pains, greatly reduced function of the lungs, coughing, extreme tiredness, difficulty with speech and co-ordination; several weeks' illness
4.0 to 10.0	4 hours	lethal dose for mice, rats and hamsters

Numerous studies show that ozone causes discomfort to people, even in minute quantities. Ozone can harm you if you breathe it in, swallow it, or by skin contact. Table 4.1, compiled by the Danish Institute of Technology, summarises documented research into these health problems.

You can smell ozone at a concentration of 0.01 ppm. At a concentration of 0.1 it can cause headaches, nausea, irritation to the eyes and a drying of the mucous membranes of the nose and throat. At this level of exposure, premature ageing may result if exposure is sufficiently prolonged. Harmful health problems will vary depending on how long and how much ozone you are exposed to – along with any pre-existing physical weaknesses.

Dust

Dust is given off by paper and toner. The amount of dust varies from one machine to another and is also dependent on the type of paper used.

The toner powder itself has been under suspicion for some time and more in-depth research into its harmful effect is currently being conducted. The initial results of these investigations point towards two substances which are chemical constituents of the toner powder: methacrylate and styrene. During the printing process, as these substances are being heated, a process of decomposing takes place which releases acids. These acids are known to be able to penetrate the skin resulting in various degrees of skin irritation such as rashes or eczema.

Health and safety rules

Control of Substances Hazardous to Health Regulations 1988

- Effective from 1st October 1989, these regulations make it the responsibility of all employers to make a suitable and efficient assessment of any health risks attributable to dangerous substances on their premises.
- It is compulsory for employers to be aware – and to warn employees and visitors to their premises – of any hazards and risks which they are liable to encounter which are attributable to hazardous substances occurring in the premises.
- It is also the responsibility of employers to ensure that all equipment is properly maintained and performs safely and efficiently.
- Employers must also keep employees under suitable health surveillance and make and keep relevant health records on each employee for thirty years.
- Failure to comply with these regulations is an offence and ignorance of responsibilities under the act is not considered as a defence. The only defence is that all reasonable precautions were taken to comply with the regulations.

Problems of heat and ventilation

Computers, VDUs, printers and other office equipment generate considerable heat. Two personal computers and a printer in a 20 sq metre office with electric lighting will generate over 2000 watts of heat. This can cause problems in rooms without adequate air conditioning, ventilation and humidification – and greatly contributes to the sick building syndrome (see Chapter 26).

Problems of noise

Noise from printers can be quite clearly heard over the clicks, hum and buzz of the general equipment in the new electronic office. Frequent or continued exposure to this noise can cause a variety of ear problems, some of which can lead to permanent deafness. Tinnitus is a common complaint, sometimes described as a fairly continuous noise in the head. Once these symptoms occur the only treatment is to completely cease to expose the ears to the offending sound; otherwise the damage will become permanent.

Other varying degrees of deafness, which occur through being exposed to noise, are caused by permanent damage to the nerve cells in the inner ear. Stress is also suffered by people exposed to excessive or continuous noise.

Sound is recorded in decibels (dBA). There is no universally acceptable safe noise level. Decibel measurement is confusing in that it rises logarithmically, not arithmetically – which means that an increase of three decibels roughly doubles the level of noise.

In West Germany the maximum legal level for noise in the workplace is 70 dBA.[28] In Britain there is no legal maximum for most sites where VDUs are used. The requirement by the civil service trade union is a maximum of 55 dBA, in any office, with the windows closed. For occupations requiring a high degree of mental effort (this includes VDU tasks) the maximum level is 50 dBA. Yet the Health and Safety Executive Code of Practice says:

If exposure is continued for 8 hours in any one day, and is to a reasonably steady sound, the sound level should not exceed 90 dBA.[27]

The British civil service union's level is exceeded by just one daisywheel printer which, alone, gives off an average 75 dBA.

What you can do to protect yourself

1 Acoustic hoods reduced the noise from printers considerably. It is advisable to ensure that an acoustic hood is an add-on purchase with every printer. The effectiveness will depend on the particular combination of printer and hood.
2 Printers should preferably not be placed in the same room as VDU operators.

3 Carpet floors and cover partitions and walls with sound absorbing materials.
4 Laser printers must be placed in a separate room or corridor with sufficient ventilation.
5 Connect the exhaust outlet of the printer directly to an external extractor fan. Ensure that the exhaust outlet is not pointing towards any permanent workplace.
6 The distance of printers to the nearest workplace – if no separate room is provided – should be at least three to four metres.
7 Detachable tightly packed granulated carbon filters will completely eliminate ozone and dust from the printer exhaust – provided the filters are big enough and properly fitted.
8 Check that internal and external filters are regularly cleaned or replaced by a reputable maintenance engineer.
9 Before hi-tech equipment is installed or used the potential heat, radiation and noxious chemical emissions should be clearly determined and eliminated, so that operators are guaranteed that they will not have the quality of their life reduced by any unwanted harmful side effects.

Other sources of noise, and related health problems, are considered in Chapter 24.

PART TWO

Epidemics

CHAPTER FIVE
International health risks escalate

Internationally, millions of VDU operators become ill after they start using computers.

Within ten years of VDUs becoming commonplace in offices, five groups of operators' health problems reached epidemic proportions. They were:

- Miscarriages, deformed babies and still-births.
- Eye troubles – causing headaches, eyestrain and cataracts.
- Skin blotches, spots, rashes, dryness and premature ageing.
- Headaches and migraines originating from stress, visual and musculoskeletal problems.
- Musculoskeletal problems (including RSI).

The puzzling thing was that not everybody suffered from the same problems. Some people appeared not to suffer at all. Outbreaks of a health problem in one company did not occur in others. Strange! But very convenient for some. Because this puzzle lent a degree of credibility to governmental bodies and manufacturers who issued emphatic and authoritative denials that any of these problems were caused by the VDU.

Secretly, using today's VDU operators as guinea pigs, millions of pounds of taxpayers' money is being spent whilst approved scientists and epidemiologists investigate the health problems in earnest. Fighting against time, they are finding ever increasing evidence of real suffering on a colossal scale. International conferences of specialists compare notes.

Part 2 of this book is concerned with the amount of suffering – the facts and figures – relating to the most common of the VDU operators' health problems.

Part 3 and Part 4 explain why and how the health problems arise and what you can do to protect yourself.

It is quite possible that even more serious health problems will emerge, whose effects take a much longer period of time to develop before their symptoms are recognisable – and, sometimes, incurable! – as were those connected with X-rays, asbestos, Sellafield and Chernobyl.

CHAPTER SIX
Problems with pregnancy

Whilst some countries forbid pregnant women to work on VDUs, others
(including Britain and the USA) have ignored or withheld available facts,
figures and research results. Will anti-abortion groups view the acquiescence of
manufacturers and governmental regulatory agencies as the maiming and mass
murder of millions of foetuses? It is unlikely that a plea of nonculpable
homicide will appease sufferers.

Official logic repeatedly concludes that the international multiple occurrences of
clusters of miscarriages amongst VDU workers prove nothing. What that means
is that, at the outset, there was no scientific proof of the *exact causes* of these
clusters of miscarriages. The scientists, bureaucratic bodies and those manufacturers who had most to gain financially said that conclusions cannot be drawn
without 'long-term' studies to support them. Nonetheless, by the mid 1980s it
was certainly easy to establish the risk that VDU users were exposed to by
comparing the incidences of miscarriages, deformed foetuses and still-births
among VDU users with those among non-users.

Whether we look at the results which are revealed from small numbers of staff in
one organisation, or studies involving tens of thousands of people, a consistent
pattern emerges. Repeatedly, the results show that unsuccessful pregnancies among
VDU users are on average around 75% more common than among non-users.

Naturally individuals are concerned about their personal consequences. Nonetheless, because there are in excess of 82 million VDUs in use internationally, and
because an excessively large proportion of those VDUs are operated by men and
women in their reproductive years, we surely must be alarmed at the yearly
prospect both of losing babies through miscarriage and introducing into the
world additional millions of deformed babies.

The results of surveys clearly demonstrate that the risk of an unsuccessful
pregnancy increases proportionately with the number of hours spent exposed to a
VDU that is switched on.

The problems began to emerge as early as 1979 in Canada.

Facts and figures

1 Between May 1979 and May 1980 four out of seven pregnant women at the
   Toronto Star gave birth to babies with congenital defects. These included
   multiple heart abnormalities, cleft palate, underdeveloped eye and club
   foot. The four women with abnormal babies worked on VDUs. The three
   women who gave birth to normal babies did not.[17]
2 At Sears Roebuck in Dallas, between May 1979 and June 1980, from the
   pregnancies of twelve VDU users, seven ended in miscarriages and an
   eighth baby, born prematurely, later died of intercranial haemorrhage.[20]

3 Between December 1979 and February 1981, seven out of thirteen pregnancies ended in miscarriages among women who used VDUs at Dorval Airport in Montreal.[17]

4 During one year, from mid-1979 to mid-1980, ten out of fifteen pregnancies of VDU users ended with three birth defects and seven spontaneous abortions at the Defence Logistics Agency in Atlanta, Georgia.[21]

5 At Pacific Northwestern Bell in Washington, USA, out of five pregnancies of VDU users during 1980/81, one woman gave birth to a Down's syndrome child, another child was born with an open spine, and a third was stillborn; only two normal babies were born.[17]

6 United Airlines Reservation Centre in San Francisco had a 50% rate of adverse pregnancies between 1979 and 1984. All of the VDU operators used one particular make and model of VDU. There were forty-eight pregnancies. The twenty-four abnormal pregnancies included fifteen miscarriages, two serious birth defects, two premature births and one stillbirth.[26]

7 During a sixteen-month period in 1982/3, seventeen out of thirty-two pregnancies ended abnormally among VDU operators at the American General Telephone Co. of Alma, Michigan. Twelve pregnancies ended in miscarriage, three babies were born prematurely and two were still-born.[26]

8 During 1983 there were six miscarriages out of fifteen pregnancies of VDU workers working at Southern Bell, in Atlanta, Georgia.[27]

9 Concern was aroused when it was discovered that since 1978, 80% of pregnant women suffered spontaneous miscarriages while working on VDUs at the public library in Aarhus, Denmark's second largest city. (We are not given the figures for birth deformities). As a result, whilst investigations continued at the library, the Clinic for Occupational Medicine in Aarhus organised a long-term study of over 50,000 women throughout Denmark. The results of those investigations should be available during 1992.[29,30]

10 At the beginning of 1982, on behalf of the British Civil Service Medical Advisory Service, Dr Bernard Lee conducted a survey of 803 women at the Department of Employment in Runcorn, Cheshire. These women worked at least ten hours per week with VDUs in the three months prior to and the three months after conception. The results of these women's pregnancies were compared to a control group of women of the same age who were working in the same office complex but who were not regularly using VDUs.

Dr Lee found that over 43% of the pregnancies in women who worked at VDUs ended unsuccessfully. Among VDU operators, of 55 pregnancies there were 14.5% miscarriages, 6.7% still-births, and 22% malformations. This compared to a 16% adverse pregnancy outcome in the control group of 114 pregnancies.

The conclusions say that 'this does not enable us to state that there is a relationship between VDU operation and these obstetric problems. The figures however indicate that *there is more than a 95% chance of there being a connection between VDUs and miscarriage.*'[18]

11 Out of seven pregnancies of women using VDUs at the Solicitor General's office in Ottawa, not one resulted in the birth of a healthy full-term baby. 100% adverse pregnancy outcome here.[17]

12 Eight out of ten pregnancies of women working with VDUs were abnormal at the Greater Manchester Fire Service. There were two miscarriages, three hospitalisations with high blood pressure, four threatened miscarriages, four emergency caesarean sections and problems at birth.[22]

13 Out of five pregnant women working with VDUs at a bank in Grimsby, three had miscarriages, one baby was born deformed and the last of the five was stillborn. No successful pregnancies whatsoever.[22]

14 At British Telecom offices in Bristol, four out of five pregnancies of VDU users ended in miscarriage during 1983.[22]

15 Alison McDonald and her colleagues from the Institute of Research in Health and Safety of Workers, Québec, reviewed 104,620 pregnant women who were classified into 42 different occupational groups. For non-VDU users the average rate of miscarriages was 5.7%. The rate of miscarriages for VDU workers varied from 8.2% to 45%. The length of time each spent in the vicinity of a switched on VDU appeared to be an important factor.

   In 586 pregnancies of women using VDUs for *less than three hours daily* the average rate of miscarriages rose to 8.2%.

   In 709 pregnancies of women using VDUs for *at least three hours daily* the miscarriages rose to 9.3%.[2]

   Thus VDU users exposed to the screen for 15 hours or more per week will have 36,000 more miscarriages for every million pregnancies than non-VDU users. Figures on malformed babies born to VDU users were not included.

16 In Finland, Kari Kurppa and colleagues investigated the cases of 490 VDU-operating mothers of *deformed children* whose birth defects included cleft lips, defects of the central nervous system, and skeletal or cardiovascular defects. This team could not find proof that the VDU caused these birth defects. Something connected with working with a VDU was responsible but they did not know what. No mention was made in this report of miscarriages or still births.[3,5]

17 In May 1986, Ulf Bergqvist presented a paper at the international conference on Work with VDUs in Sweden, summarising reports from seven different international epidemiological studies of adverse pregnancy outcomes which collectively involved 27,500 VDU workers. The average miscarriage rate of these groups of VDU workers rose to 52%, compared to a 10% to 20% miscarriage rate amongst the local populations of non-VDU users.

   Deformed babies resulted from 35% of VDU workers' pregnancies compared to only 1.4% of non-VDU users.

   The results of these tests indicate an increase of between 320,000 and 420,000 additional miscarriages per million pregnancies for VDU workers, plus an additional 336,000 birth deformities per million. That's 756,000 unsuccessful pregnancies out of every million. Over 75%. That is a lot of miscarriages, birth deformities, physical suffering and heart-break.

Ulf Bergqvist concludes his report by saying, '*VDU work has not been shown to constitute a risk of adverse pregnancy outcomes. Formally, this is not the same as stating that no risks occur.*'!

Bergqvist called for further research into suspect areas such as magnetic fields, teratogenic or teratoxic effects and stress, and for attempts to decrease the electromagnetic fields around VDUs. And he stressed the importance of good ergonomics (specially designed chairs and work-terminals).[4]

18 In a Swedish study, 4,117 female clerks at Social Security Bureaus were split into five groups ranging from those with no VDU exposure to those who had been exposed to VDUs for a maximum of not more than *15 hours per week*. This study concentrated on birth deformities in children. It does not include any details on the numbers of women who suffered miscarriages, nor does it include details of any still-births.

Group B (412 women) used VDUs for not more than 2 hours per day. From that group there was a 100% increase of significant birth malformations over the expected numbers.

Birth defects from the combination of mothers from groups A (2,748 women) and B (412 women), the two groups of VDU users, showed that 33% more of them produced babies with malformations of the heart than the mothers who did not use VDUs.[6]

To summarise the results: of the two groups A and B who used VDUs for a maximum of two or three hours daily respectively, the actual incidence of deformed babies was four times higher in group A, and five and a half times higher in group B, than would be the case for non-VDU users in the population as a whole.

Group A represents an increase of 64,748 deformed babies out of every million births. Group B represents an increase of 92,233 deformed babies out of every million births by VDU users. None of these women were exposed to the VDU for more than 15 hours per week. The miscarriage figures were not included.

19 On behalf of Kaiser Permanente, a health insurance company, Marilyn K. Godhaber researched 1,583 pregnant women attending obstetrics and gynaecology clinics in the San Francisco Bay area of California. This research found that the risk of both early and late miscarriages increased by about 80% for all women who worked on VDUs for more than 20 hours each week, compared to women who did similar work without computers.

Godhaber and her colleagues Dr Robert A. Hiatt and Dr Michael R. Polen found that the time factor of working over 20 hours per week at the screen is significant.

Amongst one of the groups surveyed – administrative support and clerical workers who used VDUs continually – the miscarriage incidence was 240% higher than for the non-exposed workers in the same category.

Whilst the researchers could not say what caused the problem, they concluded: 'This suggests to us that it is something to do with the (VDU) occupation'.[16,28]

This survey found a rate of miscarriages equivalent to 800,000 out of every million pregnancies for VDU workers who are exposed to the screen for more than four hours daily.

20 In Japan, the General Council of Trade Unions carried out a survey of 13,000 VDU workers; 4,500 were women, including 250 who became pregnant or gave birth during the time the survey was conducted. They discovered a mix of abnormal pregnancies, including miscarriages, premature births and still-births, correlated to the amount of time spent 'using' or working near a 'switched on' VDU.

25% of the pregnant women who used the VDU for one hour daily had a combination of complaints including miscarriages, deformed babies and still-births.

50% of the pregnant women who used the VDU for between three and four hours daily had adverse pregnancies.

66% of the pregnant women who had used the VDU for six hours daily had adverse pregnancies.[23]

21 In May 1986 the result of a long-term study conducted in Poland was reported at the international scientific conference on work with VDUs held in Sweden.

This Polish study was one of the first to link miscarriages and birth deformities among VDU operators to problems of radiation. Mijolajczck and his colleagues produced evidence that there was a significantly greater rate of spontaneous miscarriages (mainly in the early stages of pregnancy), malformed offspring and still-births among pregnant VDU operators than in pregnant women working as clerks with no exposure to VDUs. The adverse pregnancy rate varied between 25% and 66%.

Two different factors were found to be significant. First, it was found that there was a significantly higher number of adverse pregnancy outcomes related to increased numbers of hours worked near the VDU screen.

Secondly, they found that radiation and static levels were much higher around some makes of VDU than others. The electromagnetic field was higher around the Raytheon and Mera VDUs than around the Westinghouse models. And, the static electricity measured above the keyboards (1 metre above the ground and 40 cm from the screen) varied between 160V and 180V on different model of Raytheon VDUs, between 100V and 600V on different model of Mera VDUs, whilst it was reduced to between zero and 60V around the different Westinghouse VDUs.

As well as a high rate of miscarriages and adverse pregnancy results, this team found that other problems affecting the reproductive system were significantly higher amongst both men and women users, including incidence of infertility and various menstrual troubles.

This group went further than the numerical recording of birth problems found in other investigations at that time. Their paper drew the attention of the scientific world to the fact that VDU operators are exposed to several different types of radiation (detailing each precisely), plus chemical hazards such as PCBs (chlorinated biphenyls) at concentrations of about 80 $\mu g/m^3$, all of which occur in proximity to the VDU screen. And they explain in detail how these adversely affect pregnant women. They referred to other groups of researchers who had likewise examined the 'controversial and frequently denied radiation links' connected with birth problems among VDU operators.[7-12]

Mijolajczck also demonstrated that different makes and models of VDUs were capable of emitting quite different levels of radiation, and he showed the levels to which various parts of the VDU operator's body were exposed. Some parts of the body are more susceptible to damage from certain types of radiation than other parts.

He had also discovered that non-ergonomic arrangements (unsuitable chairs, desks and other furnishings along with the inappropriate siting of the furnishings) can also be contributory factors.[13]

22 Dr Hari Sharma conducted a study among VDU operators in the accounts department of the Surrey Memorial Hospital in British Columbia where, out of seven pregnancies, three women had miscarriages, three children were born with congenital defects and only one normal baby was born.

Sharma, from the University of Waterloo in Ontario, discovered that the VDUs used by these women emitted high levels of pulsed very low frequency radiation. This team of researchers went on to study several other hospitals who were using the same make and model of VDU and found that in every case there was a similar high miscarriage and low successful pregnancy rate.[19]

23 Concerned about reproductive effects on male journalists and sub-editors, the Newspaper Guild of America sponsored Dr Arthur Frank to investigate the reproductive histories of men. More birth defects were found proportionately among male VDU users' offspring. Male reproductive organs are far more sensitive to radio frequency exposure from VDUs because the male genitals are located outside the body.[25]

24 There were six pregnancies in women who worked with one particular make of VDU at the Douglas Library in Queens University, Kingston, Ontario. During 1984 five of those pregnancies resulted in miscarriage. Only one pregnancy resulted in the birth of a child. That baby died a week after birth with a heart defect.[27]

The effects on your body

In most countries the policy now is that pregnant women, or those wishing to become pregnant, should not work at VDUs. The Polish researchers explain that:

Between the 1st and 2nd trimester of pregnancy the hypothalami-hypophyseal-gonadal-placental relationships are highly unstable. From the moment of conception pregnancy changes the normal functioning and hormonal balance of the woman's body, which depends on a progressive functional and anatomical adaptation of the endocrine regulatory system. The adaptive processes in this system start at conception and proceed throughout the whole duration of pregnancy.

From conception throughout the first and second trimester the hormonal levels (HCG, progesterone and oestrogens) of a pregnant woman are at their lowest level. Various kinds of stress factors, particularly electromagnetic fields of radiation, can cause serious disorders responsible for miscarriage or birth deformities. These disorders may include quantitative and qualitative changes of HCG in the blood of the mother.[13] It has been found that when there is the threat of a miscarriage the HCG concentration in the blood becomes much lower than in a normally developing pregnancy.[14] Electromagnetic fields have also been found to affect secretory functions of the anterior pituitary gland, controlled by the hypothalamus,[15] which seems to be the most sensitive tissue of the endocrinal system to electromagnetic radiation.[13]

What you can do to protect yourself

To reduce the risk of spontaneous miscarriages it is recommended that pregnant women (and young women hoping to become pregnant) do not work at VDU terminals. In many countries this is now the law and women have the right to ask to be moved to other work of a similar status without a reduction of salary.

The rest of the chapters in the book detail exactly which VDU-related sources cause the problems and why they do so. They also describe the many steps that must be taken to protect fertility, virility and the unborn child. If *all* these preventative measures are taken, then – and only then – might the pregnant woman and her child have a higher degree of safety whilst using a VDU.

New test signals hope and improvement

You will recall from the twenty-four cases given above that several of those early examples occurred in telephone companies. In the intervening years most of these companies have acquired new, better designed and more expensive VDU equipment, as well as adopting improved ergonomic and atmospheric conditions and working practices. It is therefore interesting to see the reproductive improvements that have emerged in the 1991 results of one epidemiological investigation conducted into the present-day risk of spontaneous abortion among female telephone operators.

- Out of 2,430 women interviewed, 730 women reported pregnancies. This represented 882 pregnancies which included 16 pregnancies with twins. 366 of the women used VDUs, 516 did not. Only two models of VDU were used; the International Business Machines (IBM) model 4978 and the Computer Controls Inc. (CCI) model 4500.

    The rate of miscarriage for pregnancies where the mother used the VDU for between one and twenty-five hours weekly during the first 14 weeks of pregnancy was 17.2%. For those who did not use VDUs it was 15.6%. In both cases the rate of miscarriage was highest during the second and third months of pregnancy.

    During the full terms of their pregnancies the 366 VDU operators' physicians recorded 54 miscarriages, 5 stillbirths and 307 live births. The

430 non-VDU operators 82 miscarriages, 4 stillbirths and 516 live births. 10 further miscarriages were not included in these results because those miscarriages had not been reported to and documented by a doctor.

The measured electromagnetic radiation emitted by the VDUs in this test was: ELF at 45 Hz (the CCI units) and 60 Hz (the IBM units); VLF in the range of 15 kHz; magnetic flux density of the VLF fields between 9.0 and 38.0 mT per second. The values of radiation emissions at the CCI terminals were, in some cases, higher than those at the IBM terminals.[34]

Radiation itself and the significance of the different types of radiation emitted by the VDU are explained simply and fully in Part 3.

Setting a legal precedent

The first successful British case, against an uninformed and unsympathetic employer, was brought before an industrial tribunal in September 1984. The tribunal found that a woman who was sacked after refusing to operate a VDU whilst pregnant was unfairly dismissed. The woman had been employed as a librarian by the Highland Regional Council in Scotland, and used a VDU for two hours a day early in her pregnancy.

The tribunal stated that the librarian's apprehension about VDU work was not ill-founded and that the council appeared unaware of the conflict of scientific opinion on the health hazards of VDUs, particularly in relation to pregnancy. VDU operators should have the right to transfer to alternative work for the duration of their pregnancy without loss of pay or seniority.

In the event, the woman's baby died two days after being born with spina bifida.[31-33]

The right to know

Available facts and figures and research results have been withheld from exposed men and women, so as not to create a panic. Young women have not merely been allowed to continue to work at VDUs, they have been, and often still are, deliberately misled and encouraged to submit themselves and their unborn babies to known risks.

At least those who are so exposed ought to have the right to know and to make a choice, and not merely be unknowingly subjected to observation as a body of interesting, long-term research. Anti-abortion groups will view the acquiescence of manufacturers and governmental regulatory agencies as the maiming and mass murder of millions of foetuses. It's unlikely that a plea of nonculpable homicide will appease sufferers.

A word of warning

There is always somebody ready to make a 'fast buck' out of unenlightened fear and human suffering. Over the past few years a few products have hit the market claiming to protect VDU operators from radiation. For example, one is a flimsy simple petticoat made from silver-plated nylon called 'silver-lining'. It was even featured on TV and proclaimed, by the manufacturers, to be just as effective as a screen of solid sheet metal. The implication was that it gave VDU operators protection from radiation.

Will the slip protect your unborn child? Ross Edwards, an electronic engineer studying the biological effect of electromagnetic radiation, said:

It claims to protect from the electric fields of VDUs, but I know of no-one saying electric fields cause the problems. All the research points at the magnetic fields, which the garment does not screen at low frequencies (these are emitted by the VDU). Secondly, it's not much good protecting part of your body. The only way to shield yourself is to encase yourself completely with a solid conductor [otherwise known as a Faraday cage, which would consist of a copper lining placed all around the walls and ceiling, or a copper box of a smaller size for you to sit in – without the presence of a VDU or any other electromagnetic emitting device] . Currently 4,500 papers a year are being produced on the effects of electromagnetic radiation on the body.

Meanwhile, several countries – and responsible employers in most countries – now give pregnant women, and those wanting to become pregnant, the right to move to work in alternative positions within the company not involving the use of a VDU, without loss of either job-related status or salary.

Later chapters identify a variety of causes of these problems and give details of scientific findings. They also describe how to recognise and avoid most of the risks.

CHAPTER SEVEN
Eye Troubles

No other light source is so incompatible with the human eye and brain patterns as that produced by the VDU.

International surveys repeatedly reveal that up to 91% of VDU workers have been found to suffer from at least one of the VDU eye-related problems.[3,4] It is very rare indeed if anyone who operates a VDU escapes at least some of these eye-related injuries. Many other types of work cause eye stresses and strains, none nearly so much as using the VDU.

There is not a shred of doubt now that working with a VDU is responsible for causing one or a multiplicity of problems including: altered rate of blinking, blurred vision, cataracts, changes in the perception of colour, conjunctivitis, deteriorating eyesight, difficulty in changing focus from near to far or vice versa, eye strain, eye stress, headaches and migraines, irritation and itching of the eyes, photophobia (sensitivity to light, needing dark glasses), redness of the eyes, severe visual fatigue, smarting eyes, an ache or pain in the eye, sinusitis, dry eyes with an inability to produce tears, temporary blurring of vision, or tired, hot, heavy, dry, burning and gritty feelings in the eyes and yellowing of the white of the eye.

Visual problems are also responsible for many muscular problems in neck, shoulders and arms because people adjust the body into a bad sitting posture to compensate for the unaccustomed viewing distance and angle of the screen.[19] This can be very dangerous.

So too can the advice given by the British trade union Apex, who advise members that if they 'cannot position the VDU within the distance of their prescription glasses (usually 30 to 50 cm) additional lenses should be provided'. This is very dangerous advice. There must be no either/or. Simply, new glasses must be provided at the employer's expense so that you keep the screen as far away from your face as possible.

If you put your head and eyes as close as 30 to 50 cm from the screen you are greatly increasing the exposure of one of the most susceptible parts of your body to more dangerous, high levels of several different types of radiation, and of falling prey to musculoskeletal problems in abdomen, neck, back, and arms. You also run the risk of VSI – visual strain injuries.

For unknown reasons, trade unions, and far too many opticians, have determined that the ideal viewing distance to be adopted by VDU users is between 30 and 50 cm. Recently some have advocated 60 to 70 cm. In fact, most VDU users who are correctly seated on a well-designed chair will find that the distance of the eyes from the screen is at least 80 cm.

Ideally, your eyes would be tested whilst at the actual VDU terminal; otherwise, you must accurately measure the distance of your eyes from the screen, and be *emphatic* about your exact, personally preferred, comfortable working distance when talking to the consulting optician.

Recently, I had a new pair of VDU spectacles made. I told the 'specialist' optician that I worked comfortably with my eyes between 78 and 82 cm from the screen.

The optician thoroughly performed a whole range of different eye tests for any signs of inherent cataracts, or other problems, reassuring me that, he knew, there was no radiation in or around VDUs. Then he tested my sight for new lenses. I thought the testcards that I was reading were too close, but I was assured that the distance was correct – and who was I to argue with the expert? Reassured, I appreciated that my sense of distance must be impaired because of using each eye individually whilst various lenses were introduced to the heavy dark testing frames on my face.

The expensive new spectacles arrived. The VDU screen was completely out of focus at 80 cm. I slowly moved closer and closer to the screen. With my head at an awkward angle over the keyboard the screen at last came into focus. It transpired that the optician had prescribed lenses with an in-focus viewing distance of 64 cm, which is what he, in his self-opinionated wisdom from professional recommendations, considered to be the ideal viewing distance from the screen!

This guy was really into VDU specs. Another idea he had (which I rejected) was to make the two lenses focus at different distances, so that I could view the screen with my right eye and read documents closer to me on the work-top with my left eye. He assures me he has prescribed such spectacles for operators in several companies. This is not an option I would recommend to you.

What the Health and Safety Executive says

Deliberately but misleadingly, the UK Health and Safety Executive says that whilst some VDU operators do from time to time experience symptoms of visual fatigue, it is not a new phenomenon.[7] Nor are cancer or heart attacks. But when over 90% of one occupational group suffer, that certainly *is* a new phenomenon. So too are several of the specific scientific reasons why VDU operators suffer on such a large scale. No other light source is so incompatible with operators' eye and brain patterns as that produced by the VDU.

As early as 1980 Ostberg demonstrated that the accommodative mechanism of the eye does show definite signs of fatigue after a person uses a VDU.[12] By the mid-1980s responsible countries introduced new laws whereby it was mandatory for VDU operators to have eye tests before they started working at the screen and thereafter to have eye tests at regular intervals.[13] Why, one asks, did the USA and Britain not afford their operators the same concern and protection at that time? At the end of 1992 regular eye tests for VDU operators will become the law in Britain.[5,6]

What the specialists say

1 Researchers at the University of Geneva discovered that no one lighting level is suitable for everybody. Adjustable lighting levels are vital to suit

individual eyes. The VDU operator works from three light sources: the images on the screen, the ambient background light, and a task light on the work-top to illuminate papers and documents to which they refer. Because of the inherent nature of the eyes of different people, some people need 10 to 100 times greater illumination than others to enable them to perform VDU tasks as efficiently as the majority of the most efficient operators working under recommended lower lighting levels.[8-11]

2 The mains electricity supply and the difference between slow or fast phosphors on the screen affect the sweep frequency of the VDU screen (and of overhead fluorescent lights). In over half the population normal eye and brain wave patterns are measurably disturbed by the common VDU sweep frequency of below 70 Hz. To provide safe conditions for all VDU users it would be necessary to increase the sweep frequency of the VDU to around 85 Hz – and even up to 88 to 90 Hz for comfortable reading.[8-11]

3 The Centre for Eye Enhancement at the School of Optometry, University of Waterloo, Canada, found that there are measurable changes in various aspects of vision after work with a VDU. The eye shows measurable signs of fatigue after screen work. The trend towards myopia and esophoria was also observed. Changes in refraction and convergence were also noticed and attributed to the eye's demand for accommodation. They feel that more research is still needed on the relationship between the eyes' accommodation and convergence of the visual system due to close and VDU work.[14]

4 Another group of researchers examined the alarming and growing eye-related problems of VDU operators[16-18] relating to visual function and workplace conditions. They found that the frequency and severity of eye problems were related to the amount of time spent at the VDU. Complaints develop most frequently when the operator has worked at the screen for two hours. In 87% of sufferers, most of the symptoms disappear within about three and a half hours after stopping work. Fig. 6.1 illustrates the occurrences of common complaints amongst both male and female VDU users.

Operators wearing glasses, particularly contact lens wearers, report more visual troubles than any other group. There was a small increase in symptoms in people using spectacles for long-sightedness, but there was no difference in short-sighted subjects.

However there was a very significant increase in symptoms amongst astigmatic people. And spectacle wearers prevail among those who work at less than 40 cm from the VDU. Eye problems decrease in number among those people who increase their distance from the screen (ideally 75 to 80 cm or more).[15] Symptoms do increase rapidly when natural vision is imperfect.[15]

Cataract formation excluded, it was found that the number of symptoms was related to the number of hours worked at the VDU screen each day, but the researchers did not find a cumulative and additive effect relating to the number of years worked.

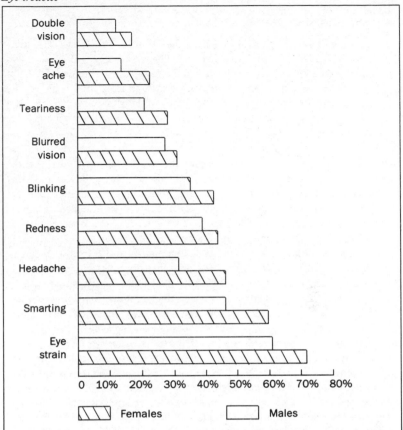

Fig 6.1 Occurrences of common complaints among male and female VDU users.

Because of the nature of the VDU screen and related tasks it was found that working at the VDU did significantly contribute to the spreading of musculoskeletal complaints, psychosomatic and astenopia symptoms.[15]

Cataracts

A cataract begins like a mistiness that develops in the lens of the eye, stopping light passing through it. It is usually referred to as an opacity of the eye. As that opacity thickens, progressively less light can be perceived by the eye. The final stage is blindness. The opacity usually develops in the lens substance itself, but there are exceptions. Some cataracts develop on the membrane which covers the lens (the lens capsule). When cataracts develop on the back part of the lens capsule, it is a sign that the cataract is caused by radiation.

In the past, workers most susceptible to this kind of injury have been pilots and those exposed to various radio and microwave radiation, both of which are emitted by the VDU.

VDU operators' cataracts

VDU operators have begun suffering from these kinds of cataracts. The most publicised cases have so far been in America and began as early as 1979 when two copy editors, aged 29 and 35, developed cataracts whilst working with VDUs at the *New York Times*. When their union took the cases to arbitration, although the US National Institute of Occupational Safety and Health confirmed that the particular cataracts were radiation-induced, the tribunal would not acknowledge that they were caused by the VDUs. The management of the *New York Times* and the manufacturers of the VDUs denied that there was any radiant energy leaking from any of the VDUs in use. They argued that whilst they conceded that the cataracts had been 'caused by something', the evidence of them did not prove that they were caused by the VDUs. The arbitrators' legal consultants used the approach that there was meaning to the 'safety standards', that the standards were absolute. Their argument was that if the safety standards were not exceeded, then there could be no causal relationship. That was a grave error.

Two years later, when an unrelated trade union insisted that measurements be made at their members' VDU work stations, they found microwave levels in excess of the safety standard. This then led to a re-evaluation of the situation at the *New York Times*, and the arbitrators reversed their first decision and found that there were, in fact, levels of irradiation which exceeded the safety standards in force at that time. (That was a permitted emission of 10 mW/cm². Subsequently that safety level was considered unsafe and was reduced to 10 μW/cm²).[1,21]

Dr Milton Zaret, a leading American ophthalmologist, has reported that the radiations emitted from the VDU include not only infra-red and the invisible non-ionising radiations but they also include ultra-violet, all of which will be more simply explained in Part 3. This was apparent from certain characteristics seen in the eyes of some patients. Some VDUs have already been found to be leaking at the frequency of the flyback transformer (about 27 MHz) in excess of the recognised (30 MHz) standard. There are also, he says, other areas which need investigation. One example concerns the sweep speeds of about 15 to 16 kHz; if there are malfunctions in those circuits radio waves can occur, and many VDUs have recently been found to emit such radiation. If parasitic oscillations occur in the VDU, energy can build up on the electron gun.

The development of cataract amongst VDU users has become more common. The first person to be actually awarded compensation by the New York State Workers' Compensation Board was a bank secretary who developed cataracts while working on a VDU. In this and subsequent cases, the people were too young to have developed common cataracts, and none had any medical preconditions to explain the formation of this type of radiation-induced cataract.[1,2,21]

Other defects

More than one third of the population have a defect in their eyesight. Many people are unaware that they do have defective eyesight because the problems are comparatively slight and do not interfere with normal day-to-day living. Working with a VDU will aggravate those problems. Undetected inherent eye weaknesses may be:

Myopia Only objects close to the eye appear in sharp focus. Commonly known as 'short-sightedness'.

Hypermetropia Only distant objects appear in sharp focus. Commonly known as 'long-sightedness'.

Phoria Most people suffer from this at one viewing distance or another, although it often goes unnoticed. It results in different images being projected on to the retina of each eyeball, the main effect being that a greater effort is needed to converge the eyes in order to perceive a single clear image at a given distance. You might squint to achieve a sharp focus at this particular distance.

Astigmatism This results in poorly focused images. It can affect one or both eyes. People are usually born with this defect and are frequently unaware that they suffer from it because what they see is normal to them. If an astigmatic person covers each eye separately and looks at an object, they will notice that the object is perceived as a slightly different shape – or appears to be at a different distance – from each individual eye.

Presbyopia This is the inability to focus close to; it is caused by ageing and happens as the lens loses its elasticity. It can be corrected by wearing reading glasses.

Anisokonia This is where the image of a given object is larger in one retina than the other, and is caused by one lens of the eye differing in strength from the other.

Problems with spectacles

Those who wear spectacles have found that neither reading glasses, which are usually made for a reading distance of 25 to 33 cm, nor distance glasses are suitable for viewing a screen full of tiny print which is usually between 70 and 85 cm from the eye. Subconsciously the spine and neck, shoulder and back muscles compensate by bending in a harmful physical manner to position the eye nearer to the screen.

Many contact lens wearers have suffered from troubles with blinking, soreness, redness and dryness of the eyes. These complaints are largely attributable to the dryness of the surrounding air because VDUs generate static electricity, and emit heat which alters the humidity of the surrounding air.

Clear unobstructed lenses in spectacles are superior to crescent or round bifocal lenses because they give a greater area of useful lens; this minimises the movement of the head as well as reducing the 'jump' or displacement of objects which occurs when the wearer looks from one section of the lens to the other.[7]

Normal changes to the eyes

Whether you work at a VDU or not, it is normal to have detectable changes in eyesight throughout your life. This is no cause for panic or alarm. But it is important if you are using a VDU that appropriate spectacles are provided to eliminate unnecessary discomfort or suffering. It is likely that you will only need to wear spectacles whilst working at the VDU and not need them at any other time. In fact it is almost always the case that spectacles prescribed for VDU work are not suitable for normal reading or distance viewing.

It is possible to have no discomfort and still not be able to see clearly; this can result in headaches and other physical symptoms merely because you will adjust your posture to compensate. Alternatively it is possible to see very well whilst still experiencing considerable fatigue or discomfort because of the intense concentration that VDU work requires; this can strain the muscles of the eyes, with a consequent increase in susceptibility to eye strain.

Eye strain is a term used to describe a wide range of symptoms including tiredness, irritation, soreness, screwing up of the eyes, photophobia (discomfort in bright light) and headaches. Eye strain is one of the biggest single causes of headaches among VDU users.

VDU operators, by the visually exacting nature of their work, are quite definitely more prone than average to the above symptoms, which are brought about by various factors, including refractive errors and ocular muscle imbalances, incorrect sitting positions, design limitations of the equipment, and unsuitable room lighting, furnishings and decorations. All these factors are dealt with in greater detail in Part 4.

As a human being grows, eye growth normally continues to the stage when maximum distance vision can be obtained without the eyes having to make an effort to focus. If the eyes' growth stops before reaching the optimum size, they will be long-sighted (hypermetropic).

In about 30% of cases, however, the eyes grow larger than the optimum size, resulting in short-sightedness (myopia), which gives the ability to see things clearly close to, but not at a distance.

Short-sightedness increases rapidly during the teenage years, but not infrequently this condition can occur in later life. Therefore the VDU operator may well attribute the cause of the condition to the use of the VDU when, in fact, it happens to be a natural development.

The eye's powerful built-in focusing system, which enables young people with normal vision to see reasonably near, loses effect with age, and reading difficulties often occur in the early to mid-forties for people with otherwise normal vision. This condition is known as presbyopia.

About the age of 45, you may be able to read the VDU display (at a distance of about 80 cm) quite easily; but difficulties often occur in reading documents 33 to 40 cm away. For others, at about the age of 40, difficulty may be experienced in reading both the VDU display and documents without a near-vision correction.

The eye cannot generally maintain a large focusing effort for long periods without strain or drop in performance. Yet surveys indicate that up to ten years can elapse after a measurable reduction in near vision has occurred before the worker takes remedial steps.

Movements of the eye are controlled by muscles attached to the outside of each eyeball. The slightest malfunction of any of these muscles or their nerve supply can lead to poor co-ordination of the eyes, with consequent feelings of fatigue, discomfort, headaches and blurred or double vision. Indeed, malfunction of eye co-ordination may cause more trouble among VDU operators than focusing defects.[20]

It is therefore in everyone's interest for employees to be encouraged to undergo regular eye examinations by a qualified ophthalmic optician or ophthalmic medical practitioner.

How to protect yourself

1 If you did not have your eyes examined before you started working with a VDU, you should do so now. Thereafter arrange to have regular checks at the intervals recommended by the eye specialist. A vision test/screen and prescriptive glasses are not a substitute for a full eye examination by an ophthalmic optician or ophthalmic medical practitioner. Pathological conditions may be overlooked and essential treatment delayed.

   You must tell the specialist that you work with a VDU screen and ensure that if prescription spectacles are required they are made for the *exact viewing distance at which you comfortably work from the screen when you are sitting with the body in a well-supported position*. Measure the distance carefully – and insist. You do have a right to take time off work for eye tests, without the loss of salary, and to use a specialist of your own choice.[5,6]

   Many companies now arrange for eye examinations to be performed at the workplace. The advantage is that the specialist can check the working conditions and exact distances between your eyes and the screen.

   ■ VDU operators must have an authoritative professional record of the condition of the eyes when they start operating the VDU and a record of what deterioration, if any, occurs in the eyes.
   ■ Any defects in the eye must be treated and/or corrected, if necessary, by the prescription of appropriate spectacles.
   ■ It is the employer's responsibility to meet any costs involved. Self-employed people can claim the expense against tax.

2 Both for the eye specialists and yourself (in case severe problems develop after some years working with the VDU) it is advisable to keep your own personal record of:
   (a) The makes, models and serial numbers of the VDUs that you operate.
   (b) The condition of your eyes and eyesight at regular intervals.
   (c) Dates of initial eye test and of regular checks thereafter.
   (d) Number of hours' VDU use per day per week.
   (e) Length of a typical session and rest breaks.
   (f) Position of display screen (above, at, or below eye level).
   (g) Position of documents.
   (h) Working distances to screen, keyboard and documents.
   (i) Any symptoms associated with VDU work (including headaches, etc.)
   (j) Lapse of time after the onset of VDU work before the symptoms occur.
   (k) The time after VDU work ceases for the symptoms to disappear.
   (l) Any medications taken to relieve the symptoms.

3 The quality of air near the VDU is important for the eyes. If discomfort is suffered, refer to Chapter 26 for further advice.

4 Radiation can be a factor involved in eye problems. See Part 3.

5 Specific lighting conditions are required by VDU operators to protect the eyes. These relate to the contrast on the screen, the work-top and the background. There is more information in Chapter 25.

6 Protect yourself by ensuring that:

   (a) There is absolutely no perceptible flicker on the screen when it is switched on.

   (b) You must have control of the screen brightness and contrast so that it can be adapted to your own individual vision and eyes.

   (c) The images and letters on the screen must be absolutely clear and sharp.

   (d) There must be absolutely no reflections whatsoever on the screen from surrounding lighting, windows, or furnishings.

   (e) There must be no glare on the screen.

   (f) The screen must be fitted with an earthed antistatic screen. Regular checks should be made to ensure it has not lost its protective abilities. Most have been found to become ineffective after six months – it is suggested that the fault lies in inappropriate cleaning methods.

   (g) Do not stand with a group of people around one screen for more than a minute or two at the most. The head, neck and body will be bent encouraging musculoskeletal problems, and the eyes are unlikely to tolerate the angle and distance of viewing without placing stresses and strains on the delicate eye muscles. Children viewing at an odd angle can be more prone to photosensitive epileptic fits if they are susceptible to them.[2] The screen is not a blackboard; it is not intended for group activities. There should be one screen for each user.

   (h) Ergonomically designed chairs and work stations must be used. Chapter 22 is devoted to these requirements.

Later chapters identify the various causes of these problems and give details of scientific findings. They also describe how to recognise and avoid most of the risks.

CHAPTER EIGHT
Skin complaints

Researchers were asked; Are skin problems related to VDU work? After their researches were completed, the unqualified answer was *yes*.

It is commonplace for people with skin complaints to find that these problems become drastically worse when they use a VDU. Enormous numbers of people with no previous skin problems before they began using the VDU have found that skin problems occur. Often the symptoms ease, or disappear, when people are away from the VDU environment for a few days or weeks.

What the surveys reveal

1 Research in Norway has revealed that between 30% and 70% of VDU users suffer from skin complaints including reddening, rashes, itching and tingling sensations.

It was discovered among sufferers that their body charge of static electricity was unusually high, in the range 5,000 to 10,000 volts. This is not uncommon for anyone working with a VDU. The static near the VDU can result in electric field intensities in the vicinity of the face of 500 to 1,000 volts/cm.

The report explains that the surrounding air carries minute chemical and dust particles each of which will carry an electrical charge that is influenced by the static in the VDU terminal. These charged dust and chemical particles get deposited on the skin. Deposition has been measured at a rate of 1,000 particles per square millimetre per hour in modern offices where VDUs are *not* in use. Under the conditions of the extreme electromagnetic fields that surround all VDUs, deposition increases dramatically and has been measured in excess of 10,000 particles per square millimetre per hour. It is not known what particle deposition rates cause the skin problems.

The report recommended that emphasis needs to be put on the quality of air surrounding the VDU terminal, in terms of humidity, ventilation, air temperature, and chemical pollutants from sprays. The researchers also say that contributory damaging effects can occur from other equipment in the terminal, particularly laser printers and photocopiers, the electrostatic properties of furniture, clothing and floor coverings.[1]

2 A second Norwegian investigation of VDU users from different companies discovered that facial rashes developed after between less than two hours work and up to five hours work. Users often described how, before the outbreak, they had a feeling of itching or of being cautiously

patted with a feather; then redness of the skin developed. Many also developed scaling of the skin and pimples. The skin eruptions usually disappeared a few hours after leaving work.

Some cases however needed more than eighteen hours to recover. By this time most of the people were back at work and the problems continued to worsen.

All working rooms where skin troubles occurred were covered with carpets of synthetic fibres except one that had a vinyl floor covering. There was a substantial amount of static electricity in all the rooms where operators developed their dermatitis. Replacement of floor coverings with antistatic carpets (with a metal thread woven into the carpet and earthed) was carried out, and this seemed to stop most cases from recurring.

In one office where three VDU operators were working the skin problems became even worse after the new carpet had been fitted. The industrial hygienist, who had conducted the environmental survey before the improvements were made, took measurements of the electrical conductivity of the new carpet. To his surprise he found that it was near zero. It was found that the new carpet was fastened to the floor with a substantial amount of isolating glue and so was not properly earthed. After replacing the carpet and the isolating glue, proper earthing was secured and the skin manifestations and complaints disappeared.

This report determined that static electricity generated by the VDU, static electric fields and airborne dust particles charged with static caused VDU operators' skin problems.[2] It should also be noted that wearing shoes or trainers with synthetic soles can also increase the static charge.

3 Mr Walter Cato Olsen and his team at the Christian Michaelson Institute in Bergen, Norway, acknowledged that the VDU terminal can be responsible for causing some operators to suffer from skin problems.

The results of a survey of electrostatic phenomena in VDU work areas indicate that rash-prone operators are commonly exposed to extreme electrostatic fields. These are caused partly by high voltages associated with display screens and partly by electric charges accumulated by the bodies of the operators.

He explains that submicron particles (particles present in the air that are invisible to the human eye and can be detected only by an extremely powerful microscope) increase substantially wherever there is an electric field like that surrounding the VDU. These, he says, cause the rashes and possibly also other health problems such as eye discomforts. Further research should be carried out in order to investigate whether or not red eyes in VDU operators might also be caused by submicron particles.

Everyone working with a VDU should eliminate the build-up of static electricity by earthing those units which generate very high electrostatic fields. The manufacturers should also design the units in such a way that the outside screen potential is much safer. Furthermore, Olsen adds, the employer should be responsible for designing the terminal so that the operator is not subject to a build-up of high levels of static electric charges on the body.[3]

4 In Canada, Dr Hari Sharma found a relationship between VDU operators' skin problems and the extremely low frequency (ELF) radiation emitted from VDUs.[4]

5 In America, ultraviolet radiation from the VDU was suspected of causing skin problems that erupted during VDU work, cleared up when the operator was away from the VDU for a period, then characteristically returned when VDU work was resumed. After extensive tests the researchers concluded that it was not in fact the ultraviolet radiation that caused the problems but some other form of electromagnetic radiation emitted from the VDU.[5]

6 Several tests on VDU-related skin problems have been conducted in Sweden.

(a) In one group, 61 VDU operators suffered from 16 different types of skin complaints including eczema, dry skin, redness, itching and/or dryness, pimples, seborrhoeic dermatitis, rosacea (chronic disease of the skin of the nose, cheeks and forehead characterised by flushing and redness of the skin, pimples and puss-filled pimples). All were subjected to a high positive electrostatic charge from the VDU.[6]

(b) Another group of 100 VDU users were examined, it was found that 22 had seborrhoeic dermatitis, 16 suffered from acne, 15 from rosacea, perioral dermatitis, 11 from telangiectasia, 8 from atopic dermatitis, 9 had only mild skin irritation, 13 suffered from pustulosis, urticaria, otitis etc. Only 6 had trouble-free skin.[7]

7 Soon after VDUs were introduced in the offices of a paper pulp mill in Umea, Sweden, 64% of the people who used them developed skin problems. All suffered from itching, burning sensations and swelling of the skin on the cheeks, forehead and chin. Various kinds of pimples, spots and rashes appeared. Only two of the workers who did not use the VDUs reported very much milder symptoms of the same kind.

It was noticed that, in most sufferers, the skin problems were more pronounced on the side of the face most often turned toward the VDU (probably because they would place work-top based documents to which they were referring on either the left or right-hand side of the screen). When the operators were away from the office most of the visible skin problems disappeared. These symptoms were not present during weekends and holidays.

The question was: Are the skin problems related to VDU work? The unqualified answer was: *Yes*.

Most of the operators had been working in this building for several years without any symptoms of this kind. The skin problems disappeared even when other kinds of non-VDU office work were continued in the same room by the same people.

Suspected areas where more investigations continued were the electrostatic field strength created by the VDUs. The original electrostatic field strength was 20 kV/m. After earthed electrostatic screen filters were supplied that field reduced to 1.5 kV/m. However, after eight months' use the function of these screen filters was checked. It was found that only

13% of them offered any protection; the remaining 87% had ceased to give any protection whatsoever. The researchers did not know why this was so, but they thought the reason might be that incorrect cleaning routines had led to the destruction of the conducting layers.

Symptoms were worse during winter, which was considered significant because electrostatic fields increase in a low humidity.

More research is needed into the question of whether the magnetic and electric fields that surround a 'switched-on' VDU can cause skin reactions.

Levels of volatile air pollutants were found in the VDU work areas of these offices which were twenty times higher than those found in another building used for comparison. Particle-bound air pollutants were four times higher.[8] Walter Cato Olsen has found that under high static fields more than 10,000 of these air-bound particles and pollutants per square millimetre will be attracted to a VDU operator's face each hour, compared with only 100 particles per square millimetre per hour when the static field is eliminated.[9]

8 Risks of malignant melanoma, the most dangerous type of skin cancer, stem from PCBs (polychlorinated biphenyls) which are used as insulating fluids in the VDU's capacitors and transformers.[10] PCBs have also been known to cause skin rashes and conjunctivitis as well as being the main suspect in cases of eczema, liver damage, birth defects and increased levels of fat in the blood – which can cause heart disease.

Norwegian medical researchers investigating the possibility of PCB leakage from VDUs in 1982 found PCB levels in the indoor atmosphere were 50 to 80 times higher than those in other offices and buildings where VDUs were not installed. They not only found high concentrations near the VDUs but also discovered that there was a link between intermittent leakages of PCBs and the occurrences of skin rashes.[11-13]

In June 1986 it became illegal to use PCBs in the manufacture of VDUs in North America and Europe. Existing VDUs were not recalled by manufacturers and many are still in use today. And, remember, the country of manufacture of many VDUs commonly available lies outside those territories.

9 British researchers from St John's Hospital for Diseases of the Skin investigated VDU operators' skin problems in a large open-plan, air-conditioned building with fluorescent lighting.

Consideration was given to several factors including static electricity and low humidity. There was a substantial amount of static electricity from nylon carpets. There was only one woman who did not suffer – out of all of the VDU workers from a mixed staff of males and females.

Their conclusion was that 'no link has been *proved* between the VDUs and the facial rashes reported. The evidence for connecting the facial rashes with the VDUs is entirely circumstantial. It is because this circumstantial evidence appears to be so strong and because no alternative explanation for these rashes has yet been forthcoming that this report is made.'[2]

See Parts 3 and 4 for the various *causes* of these problems and details of scientific findings, together with information on how to recognise and avoid most of the risks.

CHAPTER NINE
Back problems and other musculoskeletal disorders

Since the introduction of VDUs, back problems have risen by 99%, costing Britain more than £4.5 billion during 1988/89.

In Britain during 1978/79 there were 26.4 million working days lost due to back problems. The cost to industry was £900 million plus an additional £90 million to the health service. By 1988/89, after a decade during which VDUs were gradually introduced, back-related problems rose by 99% to a staggering 52.6 million working days lost. The cost? More than quadruple the 1979 figure – it was over £4.5 billion! – with over 23 million people suffering during that 12-month period. Both the number of people affected and the cost continue to increase.[1, 36, 37]

British figures on back problems have been completed up to April 1990, but at the time of writing they have not been released because they show yet another even more phenomenal percentage rise in back problems since the 1989 figures.

Regulatory authorities are so awe-struck, and disbelieving of what the present figures on back problems are telling them, that the figures are all being double and treble checked. The only increasing and significant change in work patterns, on a large scale, relates to the increasing use of VDUs.

A similar set of circumstances happened in America. According to the National Centre for Health Statistics, within a few years of the introduction of VDUs, the number of people in the US with back problems increased by 168%.

The strain of sitting

The sitting workplace has become the most common one in the industrial world. By the end of a working day many people have backaches, neck aches, leg aches or other symptoms of general fatigue. The aches and pains may be dismissed as 'irritants' but over an extended period of time they can lead to more serious health problems.

Biomechanic experts are now examining the physical stresses and strains that sitting places on the body and how the body responds to those forces. They are taking a closer look at how sitting might contribute to a variety of health problems, and how these problems might be alleviated. For purposes of research scientists tend to focus on the effect of sitting on the body's circulatory, nervous or musculoskeletal systems. However, these systems are closely interrelated in just about everything the body does.

Of all of the different seated jobs that people do, none requires the same degree of prolonged 'static' sitting as that of the VDU operator. Not surprisingly VDU operators suffer from more backache and musculoskeletal complaints than any other group of workers.

A survey conducted by the Greater London Council reflects the percentage of sufferers that is typical of international findings everywhere. It revealed that 86% of VDU data-entry operators suffered from pains in the neck, shoulders, arms or wrists. And 80% of them suffered from backache.[35] This degree of suffering can be reduced when the operators are restricted from using the VDU for more than one or at most two hours at a time (with a maximum of four hours of VDU work daily), take a regular rest break where they can move about, do a different job, walk or exercise. Of equal importance is the provision of special chairs designed for the specific requirements and demands of sitting and operating a VDU. This aspect is discussed thoroughly in Part 4.

What the specialists say

Apart from effects on cardiovascular disease, little is known about the adverse health effects of a sedentary life style. Marked disturbances in metabolism, cardiovascular responses, fluid-electrolyte balance, aerobic power and muscle-connective tissue strength have already been observed as an effect of extreme physical inactivity during prolonged passive sitting.

Some of these changes occur within a few hours or days; others are cumulative. The trend has been towards a gradual decrease in the amount of physical work performed occupationally. The benefits in terms of available employment opportunities for physically disabled and weak individuals are obvious. However, humans are equipped with a cardiovascular system, muscles, tendons and bones which have adapted to physical activity over millions of years. As the degree of occupational physical activity decreases less use is made of the capacity for exercise.

In VDU work the lack of physical activity is more marked than in any other modern task. Adverse health effects related to physical inactivity should therefore be investigated with special reference to sedentary groups like VDU operators.[2]

You might ask whether VDU operators have become the guinea pigs of the twentieth century? The dumbest animals in captivity can never be made to sit in an unnaturally static position, whether at a VDU screen, or elsewhere, even for a single hour each day and definitely not repeatedly for days, weeks, months and even years. It appears that the VDU operators have become captive and subservient, whilst being secretly observed, their health-destroying symptoms analysed and counted for the enlightenment of officialdom.

The prolonged effects

The harmful physical effects of prolonged sitting are: physical de-conditioning, decreased orthostatic tolerance, water and electrolyte disturbances, weight loss, bone demineralisation and glucose intolerance,[3-6] along with low back demineralisation and reduced disc metabolism,[7] heart disease,[2, 8, 9] lowering of blood lipid concentrations (especially cholesterol levels and LDL/HDL ratio), lowering of catecholamine concentration and effects on blood pressure and circulation,[2,10] osteoporosis,[2, 11-13] cancer of the colon,[14-16] varicose veins,[17-22] thrombosis,[17-22] pulmonary embolism,[17-22] disc herniations,[27-29] and spondylosis.[30]

Asa Kilbom concludes that what still remains to be investigated, and what training experts and employers have not yet considered, is how to make occupational work more physically active. We know that many people (because of housework, the demands of children and long journeys) cannot spend as much leisure time as they want being physically active. Moreover, it is a common observation that extreme occupational physical inactivity is seldom compensated by an increased activity in leisure time. Therefore no efforts should be saved in order to reorganise physically inactive jobs.[2]

During the rapid introduction of VDUs into many workplaces and schools we have failed to consider human anthropometry (the measurements of the human body) when designing work tasks, work stations and products. VDU users are locked into unhealthy positions and movements, which are dictated by the shape and function of the equipment. For long periods joints and small muscle groups are burdened with keeping the body or parts of the body in uncomfortable positions. The result is high local stress (which induces the symptoms referred to above).

Most jobs which were previously quite different, and had a large variation in physical stress during the day, are now carried out in the same seated and 'locked' working position in a VDU terminal. The increased capital intensity, with more money tied up in equipment, property and products, means that the work periods in front of the terminal often become long, in order to use the equipment efficiently,[17] without regard to and at the expense of the VDU operator's health.

New designs of VDUs, work terminals and working routines are essential. But the ergonomic advantages of improved design can be completely eliminated by increasing the time spent in the same position. The equipment and furnishings need to be improved, at the same time introducing a reduction of time spent in the VDU environment. Otherwise, a reduced load (stress) level on muscles and joints is counterbalanced by an increased exposure time, so that the dose of stress (load level × time) may remain constant – causing increased strain reaction in, for example, the intervertebral discs.[17, 18]

Prolonged sitting also causes a gradual strain on the heart and blood vessels, probably because of a gradual loss in the total volume of the blood, which impairs the blood circulation in the lower limbs. These circulatory changes are small and may cause no major problems for healthy workers. This can be dangerous for certain groups such as pregnant women, those with varicose veins or diastolic blood pressure above 90-95 mmHg.[23-25] Eight hours of inactive sitting causes a foot swelling of between 4% and 6% among healthy female subjects.[25] The swelling usually disappears after a night's sleep. Prolonged sitting over several years may increase the risk of varicose veins, thrombosis and pulmonary embolism in some susceptible people.

Although this view is supported by several studies, we still lack epidemiological evidence. That means large numbers of people will have to be exposed for several more years, so that we can count them whilst they suffer.

Back problems

Tommy Hansson, head of orthopaedic surgery at Sahlgren Hospital in Sweden, reports that sitting and inactivity will affect the physiology and the biomechanics of the spine in a way which can cause both acute and chronic damage to the structures of the low back. He says;

It is a well known fact, amongst the medical profession and back sufferers, that people with back pain avoid sitting and also that most back pain treatment programs ban sitting at least during periods of acute pain.

Static sitting will affect both the soft and hard tissues of the spine and will cause disturbances which can develop into both known (herniation of the nucleus pulposus or 'disc') and assumed pathological changes,[26-28] e.g. spondylitic changes.[30]

This type of physical activity will also cause bone mineral losses from the skeleton. The female spine is especially exposed to these losses because it has less bone mineral than the male spine. Even minor losses can bring the bone mineral down to a level which is pathologically low. Since bone mineral is directly related to strength of the vertebrae in the spine a reduction will also reduce the strength of and increase the risk of fragility fractures in, the distal radius, the proximal humerus, the neck of the femur or the vertebral bodies.[29, 30]

In addition to factors like age and the menopause, physical activity or inactivity are among the strongest determinants for the amount of bone mineral in the spine.[31-33] Recent findings also indicate that smoking is a powerful demineralising agent which negatively affects both the nutrition of the intervertebral discs and the amount of bone mineral in the vertebral bodies.[30, 34]

The road to recovery

In Britain, the Medical Research Council conducted a three-year trial on effective treatment and cures for back problems that ended in 1988. Sufferers were split into groups and each group was treated by different kinds of specialties within the medical profession and 'fringe' medical practices. Thereafter checks were made on the patients at intervals of six months, twelve months and two years. The results of the findings were made public in June 1990. It was found that back problems improved quicker and the improvements lasted longer amongst groups of people who had been treated by chiropractic practitioners.

I am told by Group Captain Simons of the British Chiropractic Association that official consideration is being given to introducing chiropractic practices into selected hospitals under the national health service. At this time one has to pay, privately, to consult a chiropractic practitioner.

To find out more about the identified causes of these disorders, see Chapter 7 and Part 4.

CHAPTER TEN
Repetitive strain injuries

Manual cripples blame the VDU keyboard for their injuries but radiation
could be the cause.

Experienced, fast and accurate touch typists enthusiastically welcomed the
introduction of the computer for its seemingly miraculous range of spelling,
correcting, editing and a host of other general wordprocessing facilities. There
was no problem in transferring their basic keyboard skills to the lower and flatter
streamlined computer keyboard.

Amazingly and unexpectedly, within a short space of time there were multiple
complaints from journalists, writers, secretaries, copy typists and others, including experienced keyboard manipulating experts and new operators alike. They
complained of painful new health problems affecting their fingers, hands, wrists,
arms, neck and shoulders. Identical complaints have been made by millions of
VDU operators from Australia, Canada, America, Britain, all the Scandinavian
and European countries and Japan.

These new problems could only be attributed to working with the new
keyboards in the VDU environment.

The world's fastest-growing occupational health problem

In 1985 the Australian Journalists' Association (AJA) conducted large-scale
investigations and concluded that VDU operators suffering from RSI (repetitive
strain injury) would be the worst occupational health problem in history, if
preventative measures were not taken immediately, because most types of RSI
lead to a paralysis that cannot be cured. In many offices where operators worked at
the keyboard for the duration of the working day, more than 50% of the VDU
operators became afflicted with RSI.[1]

The Australian Council of Trade Unions provided a new warning and
guidelines[2] but many employers 'pooh-poohed' the full report and ignored
completely its health and safety recommendations, just as many British employers and schools are doing today. They reckoned without the real cost of RSI.

RSI is now costing them so much in compensation claims and sickness benefit
that bosses have started to produce pamphlets jointly with the AJA to persuade
employees to be careful and to take rest and remedial action at the first sign of the
problems.

Now, the RSI complaints are recognised and accepted by the computer
industry, the medical profession, trade unions and responsible employers as
being both legitimate and extremely serious. Therefore it is unforgivable that in

the 1990s growing millions of isolated operators still do not have enough information to protect themselves.

Medical notes and reports must be specific

In everyday language these particular types of health problems affecting the fingers, hands and arms, are known as RSI. Scientists and doctors would use the term musculoskeletal disorders.

RSI is merely a convenient way of classing a whole group of health problems together which emanate from repetitive physical actions. Whilst most of these problems qualify for disability pensions and compensation there is a bureaucratic legal anomaly in some countries whereby no pension or compensation will be allowed for a claim for RSI. Operators have to be more specific and ensure that their medical notes specifically identify the specific type of RSI as tendonitis, tenosynovitis, carpal tunnel syndrome or cervicobrachial syndrome – or the newly recognised scalloped nerve endings or muscle fibres.

But such injuries are not new. They were identified in the last century and there are volumes of learned medical and scientific research papers and books on the subject. Other occupations have been the subject of RSI for a very long time and the specific complaints became known variously as cotton twister's cramp, process workers' arm, washer woman's wrist, chicken plucker's hand.

Tenosynovitis, which is the particular type of RSI from which these people suffered, has been common amongst people working in telephone switchgear, electronics assembly, printing (stripping and interleaving), small components assembly, pottery (glaze dripping), brick making, poultry plucking and trussing, meat cutting, food packing, and accounting machine operation. But there are not as many muscles, joints and tissues at risk of damage from these longer established occupational groups.

One doctor told me that 'RSI mainly happened to unskilled workers in the past, and there were nowhere near as many people afflicted from each of those occupations, which is why RSI has attracted very little earlier public attention or publicity.'

Static loading

The VDU operator's problems do not stem from repetitive movements alone. Force and static loading are contributory factors.

Did you ever play a game called Statues – as a child? The players prance around a room. Then suddenly the background music stops, or a command is given, and everyone stays absolutely motionless for as long as they can. The one who can hold his or her position longest is the winner. The VDU operator's working position is almost the same – the only parts of the body to move are the fingers and wrist, the rest is absolutely motionless for most of the time.

Static loading is the work that muscles must do to hold the body or parts of it in certain positions. It requires more energy than actual movement. You can demonstrate to yourself what static loading is about by holding your arms out in front of you and seeing how long you can maintain this position without discomfort.

Bad keyboard design

It is very noticeable that most of the workers from other occupations who suffer from RSI perform tasks which require the fingers to be in a position level with the elbow (the 90 degrees syndrome). Or, they perform their tasks with the fingers lower than the elbow.

The old typewriter keyboards had a higher upward slant than the almost flat VDU keyboard and this necessitated the elbows being bent. With the elbow bent at waist level the hands and fingers performed the same repetitive keyboard tasks at almost chest level – without any ill effects.

The hand and arm position used for the typewriter was akin to the 'arm in sling' position used by hospitals to afford the most restful and recuperative position for an injured hand or arm.

I have persuaded many VDU operators to place a thick wedge or two thick dictionaries underneath the keyboard to alter the arm position and ninety per cent (including myself) say that they have found this to be a vast improvement.

One journalist working on the *Carlisle Reporter* in the north of England, who progressed to the mid-term RSI symptoms, has found that he can ease his RSI problem by typing with two rubber tipped pencils. However, typing speed and accuracy suffer a little. 'I know it looks ridiculous,' he said, 'but it seems as if the pencils absorb some of the shock from the keyboards which have little or no give.' Those who spend repetitive periods scanning through documents and reports for editing purposes can certainly ease the painful problem a little by using a rubber tipped pencil on the cursor keys, rather than direct contact of the fingers.

What causes RSI?

All the injuries are caused by constant repetitive contractions of groups of muscles. This restricts the blood supply and deprives muscles and nerves of nourishment. Prolonged muscular contractions and the rapid repetitive flexing of fingers and wrists are the largest contributing factor, coupled with unsuitable working practices carried forward from working methods, routines, furnishing and general office procedure of the pre-computer age.

There may be additional factors involved, linking the problems to the build-up of static electricity from the screen and to radiation. At present there is a large amount of *circumstantial* evidence to support this theory but no *conclusive proof* that any type of radiation is, or is not, a contributory factor.

Operating a typewriter requires a much wider range of physical movements. Typists are obliged to bend or lean the body to take papers out of a drawer or stack, then interleave sheets of paper with carbon paper for extra copies of the work, then insert the sheets of paper into the typewriter roller, and often physically move the carriage return at the end of each line of typing. Arms are raised, body bent forward whilst arms and fingers erase any typing errors (by rubber in the early days and by correction fluid more recently). Then at the end of each and every page the arms are again raised to take the paper out of the typewriter, separate all the sheets and place them wherever required on the desk. And all this movement happens with every single page. The secretary or typist

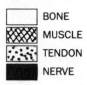

☐ BONE
▨ MUSCLE
▦ TENDON
■ NERVE

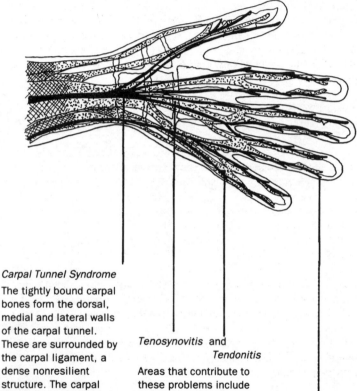

Carpal Tunnel Syndrome

The tightly bound carpal bones form the dorsal, medial and lateral walls of the carpal tunnel. These are surrounded by the carpal ligament, a dense nonresilient structure. The carpal tunnel, which is beneath this ligament, contains the median nerve which has fibres which extend to a number of muscles in the hand, mid palm, the first three-and-a-half fingers and the dorsal tips of the fingers.

Tenosynovitis and *Tendonitis*

Areas that contribute to these problems include the muscle, tendon, synovium tendon sheath and tendon insertion. If the tendon or its sheath is irritated then progressively the tendon sheath thickens causing restricted movement of the joint of the hand.

Scalloped Nerve Endings

Irritated and distorted nerves cause tingling sensations, burning, painful and restricted movements in the fingers and fingertips.

Fig 10.1 Repetitive strain injuries in the hand

might have been considered to have a sedentary occupation but in comparison with today's VDU operator she had a very physically active job.

British RSI problems began in 1982

Between April 1982 and April 1983 British Telecom performed a study of the work and motion of a group of data processors (VDU operators). This revealed that the average operator performed between 10,000 and 12,000 key strokes an hour, all day. Encouraged by bonus payments to work longer and faster, productivity of the section rose from 18 million key depressions a week in April 1982 to 21 million in April 1983. The operators worked a $37^{1}/_{2}$ hour week. The staffing levels fell from 128 to 97 operators over the same period. The VDU operators' arms never got any movement; they were permanently at that 90 degree angle manipulating the keyboard. Not surprisingly, there were an alarming number of operators who suffered from RSI symptoms.[3]

Physical symptoms

Beware of any new or recurring symptoms: you know they are not natural. Report the symptoms and take immediate preventative actions. These injuries do not occur suddenly; the develop over time and there are warning signals for those prepared to heed them.

Early symptoms are one or more of the following: tingling, aching, burning sensation, swelling, numbness or pain in the fingers, hands, wrists, arms or weakness in the muscles involved and pains in the neck or shoulder.

At a later stage the discomfort and pain can be semi-constant with bouts of pins and needles, numbness or cramps. These symptoms can occur at the end of the day, sometimes interfering with sleep. Or the operator might wake up with these unpleasant sensations in the fingers, hands or wrists. Sometimes the fingers can feel as though they are paralysed and cannot be moved for several minutes after waking up.

Finally, *irreversible damage* is caused. Pain is constant and the simplest tasks become impossible to do, like brushing the teeth, fastening buttons and shoe laces, unscrewing jars, and so on.

Types of RSI

Carpal tunnel syndrome is damage to the median nerve inside the wrist. Symptoms include a numbness, tingling or burning sensation in the palms, one or both thumbs, fingers and wrists and a weakness of the wrist accompanied by increasingly severe pain. The swollen tendon sheaths in the carpal tunnel can compress and irritate the median nerve. The problem is caused by repetitive flexing of the wrist combined with pulling and grasping with the fingers. The symptoms often occur after work, frequently during the night, or on awakening in the morning. There is often a sharp pain and noticeable weakening of thumb and/or fingers which will affect the ability to grip, turn and twist taps, bottle tops etc.

Tenosynovitis is inflammation of the synovial sheath surrounding the tendons in the hand or wrist. Caused by rapid repetitive motions. Symptoms include pain, swelling, numbness, tingling of the hand, wrist and forearm, and frequently muscle and shoulder pain.

Tendinitis is inflammation of the tendons extending from the fingers to the forearm.

Occupational cervicobrachial syndrome is muscle pain in the arm, neck and shoulders and is caused by fast paced work and prolonged muscular contraction.

'Scalloped' muscle fibres and nerve endings. Associated complaints don't all fit neatly into one of the above categories. Research carried out in Australia and published in the April 1988 issue of *The Lancet* by Dr Xenia Dennett and Dr Hunter Hall Fry reveals that they performed muscle biopsies on a group of 29 women, predominantly VDU operators, whose complaints ranged from discomfort and pain in limbs, even at rest, to total loss of ability to use a limb due to continual pain. Comparisons with the muscles of healthy women revealed significant changes in the muscles of women suffering particularly severely from RSI. Scalloped muscle fibres and nerve endings were found in seventeen of the eighteen VDU operators with pain.

Treatment and cure

There is no cure for diagnosed scalloped muscle fibres, carpal tunnel syndrome, tendinitis, tenosynovitis or cervicobrachial syndrome. In the early stages the warning symptoms of these disorders can be cured by rest. If the symptoms are ignored *permanent damage will result*, and there is still very little effective treatment for severe cases. The choices include rest, surgery or cortico-steroid treatments. Regrettably the success rate is very poor.

The Labour Research Department in London studied a group of tenosynovitis patients. The most successful treatments of the early symptoms were rest and no treatment at all. Of nineteen sufferers who had surgery, only one reported a cure and thirteen reported the surgery had crippled them permanently. Corticosteroid treatment had minimal value. Only rest and heat produced some worthwhile effects.

Hopes are raised for the possibility of help in the future. A team of researchers from Regeneron Pharmaceuticals in New York have created, under laboratory conditions, a new form of a naturally-occurring chemical that makes human nerves grow. The chemical NT-3 has been found, in its natural form, in nerve tissue in the arms, legs, eyes, brain and spinal cord. The researchers hope their findings will one day mean that scientists could use NT-3 to help regenerate human tissue that has been destroyed.[13]

The radiation factor

The greatest difference between operating a typewriter keyboard and that of the VDU is that the latter exposes the hands and fingers to several different forms of radiation that are known to have potential damaging effects, particularly on the myosin filaments in the muscles of the hands. At the same time, the hands are frequently and repeatedly exposed to what is, in very many cases, a very high electrostatic field.

Australian specialists have begun to conduct research on these aspects but, to date, I can find no scientific or medical evidence relating radiation to specific RSI injuries. Nor can I find that any other research has been conducted on this aspect.

Nonetheless, we have seen (in Chapter 8) the hazards of exceedingly high, potentially damaging electrostatic fields surrounding the keyboard. There is more information on the different types of radiation and static in Part 3.

The size of the RSI problem

- As early as 1981 a survey conducted by Western Australian Telecom found that over half the operators using VDU equipment were either diagnosed as having RSI or had recognisable symptoms.[4]
- The Australia Post and Amalgamated Wireless Ltd. has been hit so severely by huge compensation payouts to VDU operators who have suffered from RSI that it has been forced to employ a permanent physiotherapist after a 30-fold increase in strain injuries.
- In 1984, at British Telecom computer centres in Cardiff and Swindon, 76% of the operators suffered from problems in the neck and shoulders whilst pains in the fingers hands and forearms were suffered by 54.3%.
- Dr Steven Sauter, in a study for the National Institute of Occupational Safety and Health in the USA, found that 79% of VDU operators experienced finger, hand, back and neck/shoulder problems.
- Reports of surveys carried out around the world show that the proportion of VDU operators suffering from one or more RSI problems varies between 25% and 90% in different locations. There is a pro rata comparison depending upon the number of hours worked and the amount of care, consideration and money that has been spent on other equipment and environmental surroundings.

In Part 4 we detail the minimum standards of furnishings, facilities and work routines that are absolutely essential for the health and well-being of the VDU user.

The role of the unions

Trade unions have been active in investigating some of the VDU-related health problems, most particularly RSI. Internationally, some trade union organisations have contracted for their members to have their VDU working routines, equipment and facilities completely redesigned and reorganised,[5-8] while other trade unions are still lagging behind. I fear there is still far to go. This still leaves millions of unrepresented schoolchildren, as well as non-union members who are isolated by working in smaller companies and offices – often for bosses who display a cavalier attitude towards their employees' health, demonstrating a mixture of ignorance, penny pinching, and couldn't-care-less attitudes. Companies and bosses who are showing absolutely no concern for operators' health problems deserve the current onslaught of litigation which shames them – and hits them financially – in public.

The British medical problem

Gabriele Brammer of the Research School of Social Sciences at Canberra University spent four months visiting Japan, Canada, the USA, Sweden, Switzerland, Germany, Austria and England to study and assess the international experience of RSI problems.

One disquieting finding was a backlash against RSI from some medical practitioners, especially in England where, she reports, there are a disturbing number of doctors, with minimal training in psychology or psychiatry, who are claiming that these problems are 'all in the mind'.

Ms Brammer writes: 'What they are really expressing is their inability to deal with RSI. Rather than question the adequacy of their medical training, they prefer to pass the problem to another specialty.' Reassuringly, she added, 'I should emphasise here that such medical practitioners are in a minority.'[9,10]

Nonetheless, even in the minority, this calibre of doctor does exist. VDU operators confronted with this unenlightened and professionally incompetent response should consult another doctor, and perhaps report the matter to the local Family Practitioner Services Authority, the British Medical Council, and the Health and Safety Executive.

Legislation and compensation

Already legislation has been passed in some American states to ensure that equipment and working routines are amended for VDU operators. Germany has taken the problem seriously and has already introduced strict guidelines and new laws for VDU operators' working procedures and facilities. The same is true of Austria, France, Canada and Sweden.[12]

The EC is expected to introduce new legislation for employees working with VDUs. Whether this will go far enough and soon enough remains to be seen.[11]

In many countries those afflicted qualify for compensation from employers or manufacturers, and/or disability pensions from the national purse.

What you can do to protect yourself

New work schedules along with new types of desks, chairs and a host of sundry equipment and decorative requirements are essential to protect the health and wellbeing of the VDU operators. These are discussed thoroughly in Part 4. The chapters about radiation in Part 2 will draw awareness to the possible effects from those sources.

Meanwhile, the following questions point to the very minimum health and safety requirements which are absolutely essential if you are to minimise the risk to your health:

   1 Do you ever work at a keyboard which vibrates – however slightly?

2 Do you ever work with a VDU screen if the letters are not absolutely crystal clear and sharp, or with a screen that flickers at all?
3 Do you ever work for more than one hour at a time at the keyboard without then spending at least ten minutes away from it?
4 Do you ever spend more than a maximum of four hours each day working on the VDU?
5 Can you adjust the height of the keyboard to suit you personally?
6 Is the height of your chair seat adjustable?
7 Is the height and angle of your chair's back support adjustable?
8 Do you have an arm rest on your chair?
9 Can you stretch your legs to full length?
10 Do you have a foot rest or foot stool?

If you cannot answer with an unqualified No to questions 1 to 4 and Yes to questions 5 to 10, then your health is unnecessarily at risk from one of the RSI injuries.

New work practices

The Golden Rule is that the VDU operator must take regular real rest breaks away from the computer, during which time he or she must walk about and discipline him or herself to flex or exercise fingers, arms, shoulders and neck muscles. A short break every half hour is better than a longer break every hour. Likewise a fifteen minute break every hour is better than thirty minutes every two hours.

The time spent working on a VDU bears a direct relationship to the adverse health effects. It is impossible to quote all of the thousands of new work practices which have been adopted by different enlightened and responsible companies, but a few examples can be given to help find one which suits your individual office.

- At Rolls Royce and at Humber Graving Dock and Engineering, the VDU operators work for 40 minutes at the screen and then take 20 minutes off, working a maximum of 4 hours each day.
- Medishield VDU operators work 45 minutes and then take a 15-minute rest break.
- The University of Sussex have decided that 50 minutes on the VDU and 15 minutes off suits them better.
- West Glamorgan Council's VDU operators work one hour at the VDU, then take 10 minutes off.
- The London School of Economics recommend to their VDU operators that they spend 55 minutes at the screen and then take a 15 minute rest break.
- CPC (UK) Ltd. limits its operators to a maximum of 3 hours daily.
- At the Australian National University, where time has been reduced to one hour daily, it was found that 30% of VDU operators were still medically diagnosed as having RSI.
- The Berkshire AHGA (Finance Dept) stipulate the maximum any person should use the VDU is 5 hours per week, except during 'rent review' when time on the VDU screen increases to 4 hours daily.

Whilst RSI-related afflictions have been reduced by organisations whose operators do not work for more than three or four hours each day, it is not known at which point the problems would disappear altogether.

Meanwhile, it is the fastest, most conscientious and efficient operators who will suffer the most adverse effects of RSI.

PART THREE

Radiation

CHAPTER ELEVEN
Radiation

VDUs emit eight different types of radiation in measurable quantities. All have been shown to cause health problems.

Even though we are all exposed to several different kinds of radiation in our daily lives, it is only during the past few years that lessons about it have become a part of the curriculum in most schools, so it is a subject most of us know very little about. This chapter will help to give a basic understanding of where radiation comes from and why people who use computers are exposed to several different types of electromagnetic radiation which have the potential of causing a wide variety of health problems.

There are several different kinds of radiation. The term covers a collection of different types of visible and invisible electric and magnetic forces, gases or particles in the air. These originate from five basic sources: outer space, the earth, the air we breathe, all of our food and drink and man-made sources.

No-one can avoid naturally occurring radiation. Humans have lived with it in the atmosphere since the beginning of time. It is a phenomenon which mostly we do not see, hear, smell, feel or taste. But we can learn to recognise and avoid some of the health risks caused by radiation.

Occasionally I will use and explain some scientific measurements. It is not necessary to learn these in order to understand the general context. The text will enable you to understand the different types of radiation you are exposed to including those emitted by the VDU. Scientifically minded readers will find the exact measures useful.

Ionising and non-ionising radiation

Some types of radiation (which have a very high frequency) have the ability to destroy the normal electrical balance of an atom by displacing one of its electrons. The atom is thereby changed into an ion with an electrical charge. The radiation capable of this is called *ionising* radiation. All of the other types are known as *non-ionising* radiation. Until recently it has been assumed that harmful health effects could only be caused by ionising radiation. However, particularly since the mid-1980s, successive scientific evidence has shown that even the weaker kinds of non-ionising radiation also have the potential to cause some quite devastating health effects.

Safety

Radiation has to be carefully controlled to minimise possible damage to the environment and to our health. Although a great deal has been learnt about both the power and the effects of radiation, there is still much to find out. The EC laws on radiation protection acknowledge that '*no radiation exposure can be assumed to be entirely free of risk*'.[179]

Nonetheless, mostly without either our knowledge or consent, we are all progressively being subjected to increasing levels of both ionising radiation and non-ionising electromagnetic radiation. At the same time the adverse physical symptoms that millions of people suffer are counted and then analysed over many years, before new and adequate safety measures are introduced.

How is radiation produced?

Radioactive materials are made up of unstable atoms which convert into more stable forms during a process known as radioactive decay. As the decay process takes place energy is released in the form of gamma rays. The decay process may also cause the original substance to lose some of its mass, which is given off in the form of alpha and beta particles. Gamma rays, alpha particles and beta particles are the three main types of ionising radiation and they are distinguished by their different abilities to penetrate matter such as water, concrete, metals, the bodies of people and so on.

Radiation can also be produced artificially by humans; for instance X-rays used in hospitals are manufactured electrically by machines, without the need for radioactive substances. The same is true for radio waves that transmit our radio and television programmes through the air. Several different kinds of electromagnetic radiation are an unwanted by-product in the use of electrical and electronic equipment – including computers.

It is only during the past hundred years, since the discovery of electricity, that we have begun to use radiation for our own benefit. It is not only used extensively for medical purposes but also in various manufacturing industries, in agriculture and for the production of energy in nuclear power stations. During the developmental stages it has been – and is still progressively being – found that various sicknesses or death can occur to people who are exposed to certain levels and types of radiation.

We are familiar with many scare stories reported in the media about radiation-related health tragedies. To give just a couple of examples,

1 Internationally a great many early pioneers of medical X-rays suffered loss of limb and life through over-exposure.

2 During 1990 it was discovered that workers from the Sellafield nuclear reprocessing plant in England were dangerously exposed to some types of radiation. Many of the men who have worked there have been advised not to father children because the harmful radiation effects to which they have been exposed can be carried to their offspring and even to their grandchildren – now, and continually in the future.

Radiation measurements on people

The damaging effects of ionising radiation received by humans has been measured by a unit called the rem, short for roentgen equivalent for man. It takes account of the amount of ionising energy deposited in human tissues and also of the biological damage caused by different sorts of ionising radiation such as X-rays, and gamma rays.[62] Another measurement sometimes used is the rad, short for radiation absorbed dose. Because the length of time someone is exposed to a particular type of radiation is relevant (it has a cumulative effect over the years), the dose rate is sometimes expressed in rems per hour (R/hr), or millirems (mR).

Rems are now also expressed in a measure called the sievert (Sv). One rem is equal to ten millisieverts (mSv). Scientists who measure the effects of ionising radiation on people now mostly use the millisievert. Absorbed radiation is sometimes measured by a unit called the Gray (Gy).

Non-ionising electromagnetic radiation is measured in watts per square centimetre (W/cm^2). Static electricity is measured in volts per metre (V/m).

Throughout the 1980s it was estimated that on average (depending on where we live and work) we all physically absorb one mSv of ionising radiation each year from natural and background sources. However a new booklet produced in January 1991 by the United Kingdom Atomic Energy Authority (UKAEA) revealed that this figure had increased to two mSv.[179] But they don't tell us which sources have so recently caused our exposure level to double. It is most likely that the increase comes from human-made sources.

At the same time our exposure to non-ionising electromagnetic radiation is increasing dramatically, along with our increasing use of telecommunications, electrical equipment and our general consumption of electricity. For example, each Briton used 90 kilowatt hours of electricity in 1921. By 1987 that figure had increased almost fifty times; by 1987 each of us consumed 4,400 kilowatt hours of electricity,[175,176] and the figure is still rising – along with our exposure to health risks caused by the unwanted by-product of electromagnetic radiation.

Natural and background radiation

In 1990 the UKAEA most obligingly supplied us with the following facts and figures about the background radiation to which we are all exposed.

Cosmic radiation

Cosmic radiation comes from the sun, and from outer space. If you live in the mountains you get more cosmic radiation than at sea level because there is less air to act as a shield. At the cruising height of a jet you get over 100 times more radiation than at sea level.

- The average annual dose of radiation we would receive if we lived at sea level is 0.25 mSv. We get an extra .001 mSv each year for every 30 metres above sea level. For every hour spent in flight we get an extra .004 mSv.

Radiation in the air

Air contains two radioactive gases, radon and thoron, which come from the uranium and thorium in the earth's crust. As they seep into the air they disperse and their concentrations are low. But when they enter a building through the floor or from building materials, the concentration increases unless the building is well ventilated. There is a wide variation in the amount you get depending on the altitude above sea level where you live, the materials used in the construction of your building, the way that the building is both constructed and ventilated, and the composition of underlying rocks. This is the biggest single source of natural radiation. And in May 1991 the results of a survey conducted in England and Wales by Environmental Health Officers revealed that 'hot spots' of radon have now been found in an additional twenty-one counties that had previously been thought to be clear, leading them to call for an expanded survey and the provision of grants for gas-proofing houses.[182]

- The average annual radiation dose that each of us receives from the air is 1.3 mSv. In parts of Devon and Cornwall some people get as much as 100 mSv from this source because of high levels of radon and thoron in the underlying ground structure.

  If a building is well draught-proofed higher concentrations of radon and thoron can build up. This is often a problem in modern air-tight buildings where energy conservation has been a key consideration and the same old air is continually recycled.
- According to the National Radiological Protection Board more than 75,000 British homes are affected by radon. There are no figures available for other types of buildings which are similarly affected. This gas is believed to cause 2,500 lung cancer deaths a year in Britain. Scientists at Bristol University say it could also be implicated in 1,800 leukaemia, kidney and spine cancer cases.[173] In America, the Environmental Protection Agency estimates that exposure to radon gas causes 20,000 deaths a year.

Radiation from the earth

The earth is naturally radioactive. Some radioactive substances such as uranium and thorium can be found in rocks and minerals, for example granite, sandstone and limestone. As the rocks weather they form soils, which also contain traces of the radioactive materials, and the soils are washed into streams and rivers. So we are exposed to radiation direct from rocks, soils, streams and trees.

- The annual radiation dose that we are all exposed to from the ground in the UK varies from 0.015 mSv to 0.35 mSv depending on the geographical location.[63] We have already learned that levels are considerably higher in Devon and Cornwall, as they are in some parts of Derbyshire because of the subterranean minerals, granite, sandstone and limestone rocks.
- The cancer risks caused by radon and thoron are a recently accepted concern and the problems are international. In the Italian town of Aviano, fifty miles north of Venice, it has been found that the quantities of radon gas in and around the nearby NATO base are above twenty picocuries per litre of air. According to US environmental authorities the safe maximum level is four picocuries. Similar unacceptable levels have been found in Kadena in Japan.[171]

Radiation from buildings

Building materials made from the earth's natural resources like the clay, sand and gravel used for bricks and concrete, and from wood, add to the yearly dose of radiation.

- The average British radiation dose from buildings is 0.14 mSv. If you live in a house made mainly of wood the typical dose would be 0.3 mSv. If you live in a house made mainly from concrete, stone or brick, your typical exposure will increase to 0.35 mSv.[63]

Radiation in food and drink

Naturally radioactive materials in the earth's crust are taken up by plants and animals and become dissolved in water. So everything you eat and drink is slightly radioactive and your body is slightly radioactive too.

- The average annual radiation dose from food and drink is 0.3 mSv.[63]
- During 1991 scientists from Bristol University invited 1,000 schools throughout Britain to participate in the first scientific survey to determine the amount of radon in drinking water. It is suspected this could be the source of over 2,500 deaths annually in Britain.[174]

Personal sources of radiation

The body's biological systems have measurable electromagnetic properties which are necessary for the normal functions of living cells. In some instances these are measured to detect illness; electrocardiograms measure heart beats and electroencephalograms measure brain wave patterns. Additional external sources of radiation can interfere with the body's functions causing metabolic disruption of tissues and electrical disruption of cells which can have profound effects on the central nervous system.[98] The effect of additional electromagnetic radiation on children, whose bodies are still growing, is different, and potentially far more serious, from that suffered by adults. So it is also important for our health to know to what types and quantities of radiation we are exposed to.

Man-made sources of radiation

Radiation from medical sources

Diagnostic X-rays are the commonest form of ionising radiation. Radioactive materials are also used for medical examinations such as bone scans and heart imaging. By far the largest radiation doses in medicine are those used in treating cancer. A typical treatment would involve many thousand mSv, usually given as a number of separate irradiations. The radiation is carefully focused on the tumour itself to destroy it and to minimise damage to surrounding tissues. Common X-ray doses are; a dental X-ray (about 0.02 mSv); a chest X-ray (about 0.05 mSv); an X-ray of the skull (about 0.15 mSv); an X-ray of the pelvis (about 1.2 mSv); and an X-ray of the spine (about 2 mSv).

Radiation from power stations

There are radioactive materials emitted into the air from nuclear stations – and from the older coal-fired power stations (in the small particles of dust in the smoke).

- If you live close to the boundary line of a nuclear power station the annual dose is 0.05 mSv, reducing to 0.005 mSv if you live one mile away.
- The highest doses of radiation from human sources in Britain, apart from medical sources, are those received by a few people who live near the Sellafield plant and eat large amounts of locally caught sea-foods. They received 0.3 mSv of radiation in 1987 but this figure is expected to reduce as new effluent clean-up equipment is installed in the 1990s.
- The annual dose if you live within one mile of a coal fired station is 0.0004 mSv. If you live five miles away the annual dose is reduced to 0.0002 mSv.
- As a result of the 1986 Chernobyl disaster in Russia the British public were exposed to approximately 0.37 mSv of additional radiation during the first year after the accident. Radiation from the fall-out decreases with time, so the *average* annual dose that each of us received from Chernobyl in 1990 reduced to about 0.005 mSv.

  Nonetheless, in Britain, on scattered farms and on hillsides, the legacy of Chernobyl lingers in soil so contaminated with radioactive caesium that it irradiates any creature grazing on it. In May 1991, five years after the disaster, more than 700 British farms were still subject to stringent anti-radiation rules and restrictions affecting more than half-a-million sheep; experts warn these restrictions are likely to remain in force well into the next century.

The plume of radioactivity travelled more than one thousand miles to reach the UK. Clouds passed over Britain carrying the detritus of the Chernobyl explosion and rain laced with radioactive iodine and caesium poured down. The caesium came in two radioactive forms known as caesium 134 and caesium 137. The former has already decayed until, five years later, there is only about 20 per cent left in the soil. The latter will take another 80 years to decay to a similar level. The short-lived radioactive isotope of iodine has produced some grim effects. That iodine contaminated pasture, then cattle, and then milk.

The milk was drunk by children, several dozen of whom are now expected to contract thyroid cancer over the next 30 years. Yet at the time, the Environment Secretary, Kenneth Baker, claimed radiation was 'nowhere near the levels at which there is any hazard to health'. Within weeks, the foolishness of this remark was exposed – when it was revealed that radioactive caesium from Chernobyl had dangerously contaminated the animals and land on 5,000 farms throughout Britain, and rendered two million sheep inedible.[181]

Other man-made sources

An ever growing quantity of radiation emissions in the air originate from human-made sources. This consists of energetic electromagnetic waves produced electrically. These types of radiation emanate from radio and television sets and the electromagnetic waves involved in transmitting the programmes, from watches and clocks luminised with radioactive materials, and from smoke detectors and many domestic and industrial appliances. Other sources would include office equipment like VDUs, calculators and photocopiers, tools and some machinery used in other commercial and industrial processes.

- Homes, offices and factories are bathed in a fog of invisible electromagnetic radiation, commonly referred to now as *electronic pollution*. It can interact dangerously with your health and with other electrical goods. The smooth working of everything from computers and surveillance equipment to alarm systems and pacemakers is at risk. Problems range from electronic petrol pumps giving wrong prices when citizen's band radios are used near by, to stray emissions from overhead railway cables rupturing fuses in trackside circuits.

  When Ronald Reagan was president, garage doors in California were known to open and shut at will as he flew home in the presidential plane, crammed with the latest in electrical high technology.[190]
- Fall-out from the nuclear weapons tests of the 1950s and 1960s continues to give us diminishing doses of radiation which are now reduced to about 0.01 mSv annually.
- It is not possible to give a figure here for the exact exposure that any one of us receives because to some extent that depends on the surroundings where each of us spends most of our time. For example a housewife living in the country with good and controllable ventilation would not be exposed to as much radiation as her counterpart working in a modern air-

Table 11.1 The Electromagnetic Spectrum

| | NON-IONISING RADIATION | | | | | | | IONISING RADIATION | | |
| | RADIO FREQUENCIES AND MICROWAVES | | | | OCULAR RADIATION | | | X-RAYS & GAMMA RAYS | | |
	Extremely low frequencies	Very low frequencies	Radio frequencies	Microwaves	Infrared	Visible light	Ultraviolet	Soft X-rays	Hard X-rays	Gamma rays
Sources	Electrical power lines VDUs Domestic appliances	Navigation VDUs Domestic appliances	Radio, TV, Mobile phones VDUs Domestic appliances	Radar VDUs Microwave ovens	Sun VDUs	Sun VDUs	Sun VDUs	Medical X-rays VDUs	Nuclear fallout	
Medical effects	Blood disorders Leukaemia Cancer Disrupted cell growth Miscarriages Birth defects Endocrinological changes Fertility	Central nervous system effects Immune system effects Cell membrane effects Miscarriages Birth defects Fertility	Cataracts Miscarriage Birth defects Blood disorders Central nervous system effects Cancer	Cataracts Miscarriage Birth defects Central nervous system effects Cancer Genetic damage Fertility Blood disorders	Cataracts	Eye fatigue Eye strain Photosensitive epilepsy	Skin cancer Cataracts Premature ageing	Genetic damage Cancer Miscarriage Premature ageing Birth defects Fertility	Death	Death

This chart shows a summary of where scientific research has linked a health problem to a specific source of radiation tight city office block, surrounded by hi-tech equipment. Nonetheless, it was estimated by the NRPB in 1988 that the average amount of radiation that each of us is subjected to from background exposure from non-medical human-made sources is 0.8 mSv each year.[63]

Do bear in mind when interpreting these figures that; (a) the mSv is referring only to ionising types of radiation that we are exposed to, (b) our exposure to ionising radiation has doubled since these figures were released, and (c) there are no figures available to advise us how much (and what types of) additional *non*-ionising radiation we are exposed to.

■ If a person sat close to a radiation emitting device repeatedly for several hours daily then that person would be exposed to a much greater level of radiation. And remember, the effects of exposure to radiation are cumulative over the years.

Man-made electromagnetic radiation

The types of radiation made and used by humans are an unwanted by-product inherent in the production and use of a wide variety of electrical and electronic products and services. This type of radiation is collectively called electromagnetic radiation.

Electric and magnetic fields

These electromagnetic waves, mostly invisible to the human eye, travel through space at approximately 186,000 miles per second (the speed of light). They are made up of two fields (electric and magnetic) which vibrate at right angles to each other. Each has the potential to cause harmful health effects. Both fields are measured separately. The electric field is measured in volts per metre (V/m), the magnetic field strength is measured in ampères per metre (A/m), and a unit of measure called the tesla is used to measure the magnetic flux density.

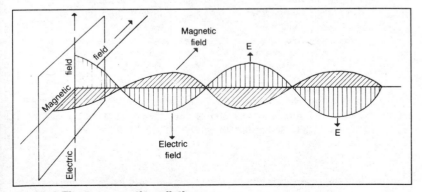

Fig 11.1 Electromagnetic radiation

Frequency and wavelength

The wavelike motion of these types of travelling energy is timed and measured according to the number of times it goes up and down each second (the frequency).

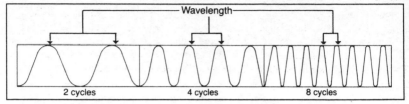

Fig 11.2 How frequency and wavelength are related

The number of these cycles per second is measured in units of hertz (Hz). A frequency of one hertz represents one cycle per second. The measurements used to identify frequency are:

Table 11.2 Units of frequency

Abbreviation	Unit	Equivalent
Hz	hertz	1 cycle per second (cps.)
kHz	kilohertz	1,000 cps.
MHz	megahertz	1,000,000 cps.
GHz	gigahertz	1,000,000,000 cps.

The length of the electromagnetic waves can also be measured from the peak of one wave to the peak of the next (wavelength).

The units of measure used to do this are:

Table 11.3 Units of wavelength

Symbol	Unit	Equivalent
m	metre	100 centimetres (cm)
cm	centimetre	.01 of a metre (m)
mm	millimetre	.1 cm
μ	micrometre	.0001 cm
nm	nanometre	.0000001 cm
A	angstrom	.00000001 cm

Frequency and wavelength are related. The shorter the wavelength the greater the frequency. For example a frequency of one hertz (one cycle per second) is equal to a wavelength of 300 million metres (186,000 miles).

Wave amplitude

The height of the peaks and troughs in the cycle determines the degree of energy and power that electromagnetic waves can have. This power level of radiation is known as its wave amplitude. This is similar to the relationship between the wattage (power) of a light bulb, the intensity of the light which it gives off, and the distance it will light up. A 100 watt bulb gives off more light and reaches further into dark corners than a 40 watt bulb. The frequency of both light bulbs is the same but the 100 watt bulb will give off a brighter light.

The units used to express measures of power differ for different forms of radiation and particular frequencies. Those we are particularly interested in, because they are emitted by VDUs, are given in Table 11.4.

Table 11.4 Measurements of power for different frequencies

Types of radiation	Unit of measurement
X-rays	millisieverts per hour (mSv/hr)
ultraviolet infrared microwaves radio frequencies very low frequencies extremely low frequencies	watts per square centimetre (W/cm²)
static electricity	volts per metre (V/m)

Beginning at a frequency of 1Hz (one cycle per second) is a band of extremely low frequencies (ELF), followed by very low frequencies (VLF), followed by radio frequencies (RF), microwaves (MW), infrared (IR), visible light (VL), ultraviolet (UV), X-rays and gamma rays. With the exception of gamma rays all of these other types of radiation are emitted by VDUs.

Time and distance are important factors

The power or intensity of electromagnetic radiation drops off with increasing distance from the source. This distance/power relationship is called the inverse square law because the received intensity falls off by the square of the distance from the source. So the proximity of our bodies to the source of radiation and the length of time that we stay there will determine the amount of radiation that we are exposed to. This is one of the main reasons why the VDU operator's circumstances are unique and hazardous.

Eight types of electromagnetic radiation produced in the VDU

■ *X-rays* are given off as a secondary emission from the impact of high speed electrons on the viewing screen, and from the electrodes of the beam gun. If the anode voltage exceeds the maximum voltage rating of

(a) The sources of radiation

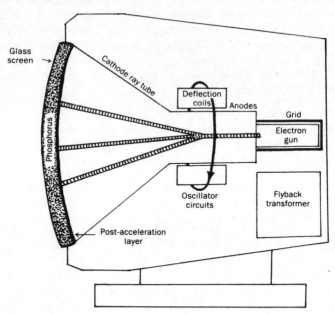

(b) Types of radiation emitted

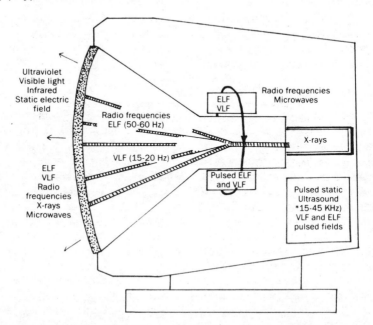

Fig 11.3 Radiation emissions

the tube, X-rays can leak through the neck of the tube.[79] Emissions of X-rays are usually stronger in colour tubes.

- *Ultraviolet radiation and visible light* are given off from the excitation of the phosphors on the inner surface of the screen. The ultraviolet should be absorbed by the glass.
- *Infrared radiation* is produced from the heat generated on the viewing screen by the impact of electrons on the phosphors.
- *Microwaves* are produced by the sweep oscillator circuits at the back of the cathode ray tubes.
- *Radio frequencies* up to 11 mHz are generated by the electrical pulses which cause the beam to go on and off eleven million times a second. Radio frequencies are also generated by pulsations coming from the oscillator circuits.
- *Extremely low frequencies (ELF)* between 50 to 60 Hz are produced from the electrical pulses which cause the beam to move vertically in order to refresh the full frame on the screen 30 or 60 times a second.
- *Very low frequency fields (VLF)* at 15 to 20 kHz are generated by electrical pulses used to move the beam horizontally 15,000 to 20,000 times each second.
- *Static electricity* is also produced as a result of the electrical power used to operate the device and also from the electron beam which is directed on to the screen. Static is also produced by the flyback transformer.[60]

Pulsed ELF and VLF

These frequencies consist of the pulsed waveform electric field from the flyback transformer lead and the saw-tooth waveform magnetic field from the deflection yoke of the VDU.

There are three major sources of these electromagnetic waves in the VDU. (See Fig. 11.4).

1 First are the extremely low frequency (ELF) emissions resulting from the 120 or 240 volt, 50 or 60 Hz a.c. input power and the vertical sweep circuits. These vertical sweep circuits, along with the wiring, power transformers and a.c. rectifiers within the display terminal, emit both electric and magnetic fields of 50 to 60 Hz frequency and associated harmonics of diminishing strengths.

2 Covering the very low frequency (VLF) to low frequency (LF) range of approximately 15 to 200 kHz is the horizontal deflection system which causes the electron beam in the cathode ray tube to sweep rapidly back and forth across the fluorescent screen. The electronic sweep circuits of the VDU send pulses of electric current through the primary winding of the flyback transformer and the magnetic coils surrounding the neck of the tube. This causes high voltage pulses at a rate from 15,000 to 30,000 times per second. The flyback transformer voltage pulses reach a level of 15,000 to 40,000 volts by the flyback transformer secondary winding. The pulses produce d.c. voltage for accelerating the electrons emitted by the tube to the high speeds necessary for visible light to be produced when

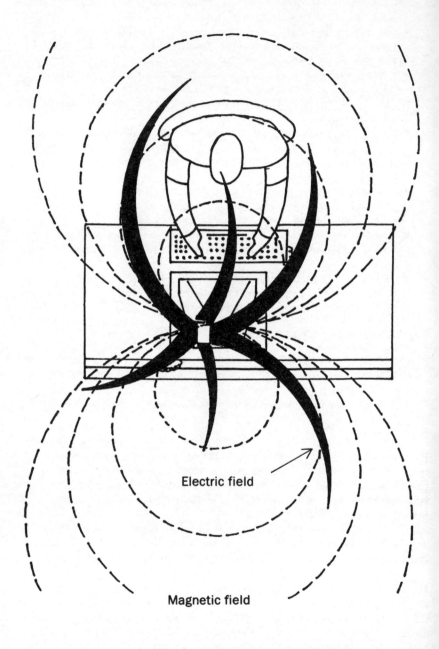

Electric field

Magnetic field

Fig 11.4 Electric and magnetic fields

they strike the fluorescent screen. This d.c. voltage is the second source of electric field from the VDU. Because of the pulsating nature of the electromagnetic fields their frequency varies from 15 to 30 kHz with significant harmonics up to approximately 200 kHz.

3 The major source of the *magnetic field* is the magnetic deflection coil. The strength of the magnetic field outside the casing of the VDU will depend on the distance from the magnetic deflection coil: it is about 5 ampères per metre (A/m) at the surface of the VDU, and is expected to fall to 0.1 A/m at a normal viewing distance.

The main source of the *electric field* is the high voltage winding and high voltage output lead of the flyback transformer. The strength of these electric fields outside the body of the VDU will depend on the location of the flyback transformer and on the amount and thickness of the metal shielding between the flyback transformer and the VDU's outer cover. Those VDUs which have metal or conductive cases will emit considerably less than those with plastic covers.[159] The electric field is commonly as high as 40,000 volts per metre (V/m) at the surface of the VDU, but is expected to fall to less than 10 V/m at a normal viewing distance.

When an oscillating magnetic/electric field passes through a conducting material, it induces electric currents. The human body is conductive; therefore any field passing through the body will induce small electric currents. Any harmful effects to VDU operators would be due to these currents. The position and angle of the body in relation to the electromagnetic field will be important in determining which of the body's organs might be affected.[180]

Therefore the effect on VDU operators will be dependent on their position, posture, size and possibly the type of footwear, as well as the conductivity of the surrounding furniture and floor coverings.[139]

Pulsed static

Pulsed static coming from the flyback transformer (usually located at the back corner of the terminal) has been found to be particularly high. This will affect persons sitting behind the VDU. A person sitting 1.2 metres from the rear corner will experience the same field as a person sitting in front of the VDU just 30 cm from the screen.

Safety levels

Understood in terms of recommended safety levels, the field strengths given above mean that the exposures at the surface of the VDU are well in excess of even the maximum recommended safety levels but, because of the fall of power with distance, regulatory bodies expect that they will be below the present recommended safety levels at the normal viewing distance.

There is growing concern in some scientific circles that the pulsating nature of the currents in the ELF, VLF and static electric fields which are generated in the

VDU are an important factor not taken into consideration when examining operators' health problems.

However, we are still in the early days for research into the health hazards and safe levels of exposure from these pulsed electromagnetic fields. The current safety standards and working practices will most probably be amended, in time – just as those for X-ray exposure have been, as you will see in the next chapter.

Call for mandatory declarations of radiation levels

Some irresponsible VDU manufacturers, suppliers and their service and maintenance engineers do not have the necessary collection of equipment to test for all types of radiation emanating from the equipment which they are selling, servicing and maintaining, particularly in the microwave and radio frequency wave bands.

Far too many manufacturers don't even know the luminance of their screens. That is illegal in Britain, where section 6 of the Health and Safety at Work Act places a duty on manufacturers, designers and suppliers to give comprehensive information on VDU equipment and also to carry out research, tests and examinations so that they know what is involved in their equipment. [107]

Hopefully – as should be the case – one day in the future manufacturers will be held responsible for printing precise details (on labels attached to all of their products) of the different types and strengths of radiation which their products emit – just as food manufacturers and suppliers now must list all the ingredients in their products.

A letter to your local member of parliament may help to bring into sharper focus the problem of increasing, unhealthy – if invisible – pollution of electronic smog in our homes and workplaces.

The remaining chapters in Part Three reveal details of scientific evidence for the health risks that each type of electromagnetic radiation has been found to cause, with advice on what you can do to protect yourself. Unfortunately this is *not* the same thing as telling you that you can completely eliminate *all* of the possible health risks attributable to electromagnetic radiation from the VDU.

CHAPTER TWELVE
Early warning signs denied and ignored

Historically, the international standards that were set for a safe level of exposure to radiation have often been proved dangerously too high. The occupational exposure standard for some types of electromagnetic radiation in some eastern European countries and the Soviet Union is 1,000 times lower than the occupational exposure standard in western Europe, the USA and Britain.

Introducing computers to the mass market

Margaret Thatcher declared 1982 to be Information Technology Year in Britain. Under the chairmanship of Kenneth Banker the IT 82 Committee was formed. Its purpose was to introduce the new hi-tech age to the public and particularly to encourage the business community to abandon old tried and tested methods in favour of a new age of computers and robotics. Representing the British Institute of Management in the north-west of England, I was a member of that committee.

The dawning of a revolutionary new age was quite exciting. Computers and robotics almost miraculously performed innumerable fascinating jobs quickly and – mostly – efficiently and none more dramatically than producing and transmitting information via the computer.

All of this was promoted, largely at the taxpayers' expense, to a population who were pre-conditioned to acquiring something new. Advertising and marketing men use the key word *new* in advertisements to sell us products from detergents to cars to seasonal fashions. Some of the new technology generated an acquisitive desire in those who could afford to buy it. Certainly the idea of something revolutionary and new generated no suspicion or fear of health risks. The only dissenters were the trade unions who were fearful of losing jobs for their members because it appeared that computers could do so much with so little labour.

Health risks ignored

Personal safety and wellbeing were neither mentioned nor considered by the members of the IT 82 Committee – or at that time by the trade unions. Officialdom clearly *assumed* that there would be no dangers to operators' health and wellbeing, nor that entirely new working procedures, office planning and furnishings would be absolutely essential to safeguard their health. Nor that the cost of the new equipment was only the beginning of the expense required when installing computers! In fact if employers, schools and home users are to take adequate steps to protect the wellbeing of operators the *additional cost involved would be at least between double and triple* the cost of the hardware and software.

Official safety recommendations

Assumptions about safety levels have been mostly based on knowledge of other industries whose workers' situation is not the same as that of the VDU operator. Adequate comprehensive research into possible health problems for the operators' specific radiation exposure levels and working environments had not been conducted. In many wavelengths there simply is still not the equipment available to carry out such tests accurately, or at all.[61]

The recommended safety levels in force today have been arrived at by major international groups working on results of tests from bomb survivors at Hiroshima and Nagasaki, from groups of patients given large doses of radiation for medical purposes and from observations and tests on workers in other industries who are known to be exposed to different types of radiation in quite different circumstances.

These groups include the International Commission on Radiological Protection (ICRP) and the United Nations Scientific Committee on Effects of Atomic Radiation (UNSCEAR). The American National Academy of Science's Committee on the Biological Effects of Ionising Radiation (BEIR) have calculated the risk of fatal cancer following a given dose of radiation.[64]

Historically the international standards that were set for what was considered, at that time, to be a safe level of exposure to radiation have often been proved dangerously too high.

Published research papers show that there has been a vast difference of opinion, amongst scientists, about what is considered to be a safe level for each of the different types of radiation emitted by VDUs. Radiation levels considered to be safe in some countries would be considered dangerous in others. For example the occupational exposure standard, for some types of electromagnetic radiation, in some eastern European countries and the Soviet Union is between 100 and 1,000 times lower than the occupational exposure standard in Britain.[65-67, 131]

Some radiation levels which have been considered to be safe in the past have subsequently proved not to be safe – resulting in amended lower recommended safety levels being introduced.

Often, where there is no previous experience of public exposure in given circumstances to a given type of radiation – or of exposure to a combination of different types of radiation – scientists and regulatory agencies use the acronyms ALARP and ALARA as the standards for exposure – until further evidence comes to light. These simply mean: As Low As Reasonably Practicable, or, As Low As Reasonably Achievable, respectively – when it is socially and economically viable!

People who felt the regulatory bodies would never allow workers or the public to be exposed to anything which was not tried and tested to be absolutely safe are now realising that, as we approach the twenty-first century, we appear to have a system where the work force and the public at large are increasingly the guinea pigs for new processes. 'New' is suddenly not as appealing to the purchaser and marketing people as the little used phrase 'tried and tested'. Table 12.1 shows the ever-changing recommended exposure levels for X-rays being continually revised and reduced.

Table 12.1 Changing international exposure standards for X-rays

1900	10 rems daily
1925	52 rems yearly
1934	36 rems yearly
1950	15 rems yearly
1957	5 rems yearly
1991	Standard now under review again!

Early warning signs of health risks

Before 1982 there were already early warning signs of possible radiation dangers to operators of VDUs. There had been assorted health complaints from operators in Australia and America where computers had been introduced earlier. There had been only an uncomprehensive and inadequate number of tests conducted on fewer than 500 VDUs. Those tests were made variously in Britain and the United States.

VDUs subjected to testing were largely being checked for emissions of ionising radiation, particularly X-rays, because it was acknowledged that this could be dangerous to health. At that time it appears to have been mostly assumed that non-ionising radiation would not cause any health risk.

A test of 115 VDUs in America in 1977 showed that 70 emitted levels of X-rays 70% above recommended safety levels.[68]

In another series of tests conducted by the Winchester Engineering and Analytical Centre (WEAC) at Winchester, Massachusetts for the US Food and Drug Administration's Bureau of Radiological Health, tests were carried out on a broader radiation spectrum, including tests for X-ray emissions, magnitude of electric and magnetic fields at microwave and other radio frequencies, ultrasonic emissions and ultraviolet and visible light radiation.

WEAC reported that of the 48 manufacturers then making VDUs in America, only 15 submitted machines for testing. The other 33 companies did not submit their products for testing – and there was no statutory requirement for them to do so. Of the equipment which was submitted, 8% gave off high levels of X-rays in excess of the recommended safety levels.

The WEAC qualified their report when they stated:

There are no performance standards setting permissible radiation levels for VDUs. Therefore test results had to be compared to occupations standards or to performance standards for other products.

Some of the dangerous VDUs were recalled by the manufacturers for modification, while other manufacturers were not allowed to sell their VDUs on the American market.[55, 56]

These tests revealed a leakage of X-rays from the cathode ray tube far above accepted safety standards. But the warning signals were ignored. The official conclusion by regulatory bodies was that these contraventions of safety standards resulted from manufacturing defects or from faults in the mains electricity supply; or that the original measuring equipment must have been faulty.[49-53]

A group of Japanese scientists put the controversy about VDU radiation emissions into perspective when they said that 'scientists who cannot detect any of the radiation emanating from VDUs are either using inadequate or faulty measuring equipment, or they are lying.'

Nonetheless, in a blaze of IT 82 publicity by the UK government and computer manufacturers, the public were encouraged to buy – without delay.

Profits versus health

Quite recently, one British manufacturer was refused permission to sell VDUs on the American market because they did not reach American standards. A metal plate was not earthed and the VDU emitted radio frequencies that could interfere with next door's TV, and with hospital equipment and aircraft controls. Those machines were sold on the British market. Others which suffer from some of the same problems could be on sale today.

Sales worth £ billions have been made in the decade which followed IT 82 by manufacturers whose main consideration is high profits. There has been and continues to be a price war, particularly at the cheaper end of the market, which has led some unscrupulous manufacturers to cut safety corners in order to cut prices.

There is no mandatory regulation for manufacturers to have the radiation emissions of their VDUs tested for safety before they are sold to the public – though new legislation is to be introduced by the end of 1992 which will make manufacturers and managements installing VDU equipment responsible and accountable.

By the beginning of 1990 it was estimated that, internationally, over 82 million VDUs had been sold. If each VDU is only used by one operator and if only 8% emit dangerous levels of radiation (the smallest number of VDUs found with radiation emissions above the safety levels in any of the tests referred to above) then that means that today a minimum of 6,650,000 people are being exposed to a dangerous level of at least one kind of radiation. And that does not take into account the fact that many VDUs are used by several different people, particularly in schools, or the combined effects of the different types of radiation and environmental factors to which operators are exposed at the same time and for prolonged periods.

It is true that if all machines were manufactured – and maintained – to perfect standards then the levels of all types of radiation emitted by VDUs 'should' fall within the currently accepted safety levels in force today. Most of the different types of radiation which do emanate from VDUs 'should' therefore pose no threat – to the average healthy VDU operator working in an ergonomically designed VDU terminal which is subject to regular maintenance checks. The exception is some of the lower frequency electromagnetic fields. Regrettably, in the real world there are few VDU users blessed with a combination of these perfect personal and environmental conditions.

VDU operators have been deliberately misled

Everybody who uses a VDU is exposed to the eight different types of electromagnetic radiation detailed above, yet this fact is repeatedly and irresponsibly denied by manufacturers, managements, doctors and even by regulatory bodies who are responsible for safety in working environments as well as for the general public in their day to day lives.

Officially, a collection of misleading statements are repeatedly made which misrepresent the true position, aiming to lull VDU operators into a false sense of security.

When being reassured by officialdom that there is no danger of leaking radiation from VDUs, the operators must learn to interpret the exact words which they hear or read – and not assume that those words mean something else simply because of the self-assured tone of voice and the assertive and authoritative manner with which they are used. For example, common misleading statements include:

- 'We *do not consider* that there is any danger' does not mean 'There is no danger'.
- 'It is *not felt* that there are any risks' neither says nor means 'There are no risks'.
- 'It is *unlikely* there would be any adverse effects' does not mean there are none.
- '*I wouldn't imagine* there is a problem.' Imagine! What about facts?
- 'No *scientific* evidence' means we choose to disregard facts and figures of suffering produced by epidemiologists if they have not been comprehensively explained scientifically.
- 'From *available* research there is no reason to believe there could be a health problem'. But they seldom add that this is because no comprehensive medical and scientific research has been completed or even begun into many suspected dangerous aspects of the VDU operator's problems. These particularly include the lower frequency electromagnetic fields, and the VDU operator's unique circumstances of being so physically close to the source of radiation for prolonged periods of time – repeatedly.

Many scientists feel that some areas of extremely low frequency radiation still cannot be measured adequately because, as yet, very few methods of accurate measurement have been developed. This is because the electrical instruments used to measure emissions can interfere with and distort the frequencies which they are measuring.[61]

The Health and Safety Executive's employees' guide *Working with VDUs* says that 'The NRPB *do not consider* that the emissions from a VDU will put either you or your unborn child at risk'. (My emphasis.) It goes on to explain that X-rays emitted from a VDU do not add significantly to the natural background level, etc.

This does not mean that working with VDUs *will not* put either you or your unborn child at risk: *do not consider* and *will not* have very different meanings.

In any case, not one of the women who have miscarried or suffered from other complaints whilst working with VDUs has accused X-rays in particular as the cause of their problem. What they are saying – and what some responsible bodies are saying who have conducted research involving hundreds of thousands of VDU operators – is that *something* in the VDU terminal appears to have caused the miscarriages and other health problems.

I posed some questions to the National Radiological Protection Board (NRPB). I asked,

'Is it possible that radiation emanating from VDUs could detrimentally affect the operators' health?'

The NRPB spokesman answered:

'There is more radiation emitted from hair dryers, food mixers and electric blankets than there is from a VDU. We don't think there is anything to worry about.'

I persisted:

'There are numerous cases reported concerning many tens of thousands of women who worked with VDUs having miscarriages. These reports come from various parts of Britain and from many other countries where working with VDUs is considered responsible for miscarriages amongst pregnant women.'

I was authoritatively assured:

'We *do not consider* that X-ray emissions from VDUs are dangerous at all. X-rays from VDUs are lower than background radiation. X-rays from VDUs are not high enough to cause miscarriages.'

I had never mentioned X-rays. I asked a more direct question.

'Will you *absolutely guarantee* that working with VDUs *will not* put either VDU operators or their unborn child at risk?' The answer from the NRPB spokesman in Leeds was:

'We *cannot guarantee* that it won't. In the light of further research something might be found. But, it is *not expected* that it would.'

It would have been far more productive and beneficial to VDU operators if the time and money spent denying the problems exist had been directed into solving them. During the past decade, when a great deal of research has been conducted and many answers have been found to alleviate the health problems, this mounting knowledge should at least be made available to the VDU operators so that the benefit of the many solutions which have been found could be put into practice. Operators could then take the necessary steps to protect themselves, rather than being exposed as guinea pigs to a repeated deterioration in health and quality of life, or have the choice of whether or not they wish to continue working with a VDU under their present conditions.

New laws and reduced levels of radiation in future

A conference which brought together many of the world's leading scientists investigating the health problems relating to VDUs was held in Sweden in 1986. One of the facts revealed was that non-ionising radiation from the VDU screen often reached a magnetic field strength of 200 milliteslas and that a number of adverse health problems could result.

Thereafter Sweden and Denmark began demanding lower radiation levels from their VDU screens insisting upon a magnetic field strength of not more than 20 milliteslas. To meet these new specifications Ericsson's VDUs (manufactured by the Noika Group in Finland, who are Europe's leading VDU suppliers) use a higher than normal refresh rate for their screens. They use a frequency of 70 Hz. Other manufacturers use frequencies of around 4 to 20 Hz, which are close to those from the brain's own carrier frequency. Taxan also began to produce lower radiation screens. Both reduced the X-ray emissions to less than 0.5 mR/hr, the magnetic fields to less than 25 mT/s and electrostatic to less than 500 V/m.

By the beginning of 1990 IBM, usually one of the most responsible and quality conscious of computer manufacturers, cut radiation emissions from the VDU screens of their newest large computer terminals, saying that they would make similar changes (at an unspecified date in the future) to their personal computers. However, they do not intend to recall or alter any of their existing computer screens because they insisted that the old levels of radiation were not a *serious* health hazard.

The British Health and Safety Executive have participated in European Community negotiations for a new directive on display screen equipment which is the forerunner of legislation imposing new minimum health and safety standards for VDU users. This directive was adopted at the end of May 1990, despite a House of Lords select committee advising its rejection in 1989, and all EC member states will have to implement it by the end of 1992. It requires employers to analyse work stations and remedy all the health risks found – to ensure that VDU terminals meet minimum new health and safety requirements.

In the UK the directive is likely to be implemented by the introduction of new regulations on display screen equipment made under the Health and Safety at Work Act 1974.

CHAPTER THIRTEEN
X-rays

The measurements of X-rays emitted by VDUs can differ considerably from one manufacturer to another and between different machines from the same manufacturer.

In Canada, the United States and Britain, the current safety standard in force for a person being exposed to X-rays from VDUs is 0.5 mR/hr, or 0.5 Sv for the body, except for eye exposure. The standard for eye exposure is reduced to 0.15 Sv. These standards were set to govern the maximum amount of X-rays that a person should receive when watching TV sets used in the home. They have never been revised for people who spend considerably longer periods of time sitting close to the VDU screen. By comparison, the national safety standard in Sweden is far lower at 5 mSv.[74] In Britain the safety levels are covered under British Standard BS415.[75]

VDUs are designed so that the soft X-rays which they generate are mostly inside the cathode ray tube, specifically the inside of the fluorescent viewing screen.[73] These soft X-ray emissions are effectively shielded by the glass screen and should not affect the operator so long as the manufacturer uses sufficiently absorptive glass for the screen and the VDU is of sound construction. Thereafter it is important that the VDU is well maintained and regularly serviced since problems are likely to develop with age.

Measurements resulting from intensive testing for X-ray emissions on tens of thousands of VDUs in Austria, Canada, Italy, Sweden, Britain and the United States reveal that whilst sensitive measuring equipment shows that the measurements can differ considerably from one manufacturer to another and between different machines from the same manufacturer, the X-ray emissions from *most* of the VDUs tested are lower than the present exposure standards.[73] But 'most' does not mean 'all': according to the Radiation Safety Corporation of Palo Alto, California, 'a recent Food and Drug Administration study found that one out of twelve computers emitted X-rays in excess of the federal safety limits'. VDUs that do not have the ability to display a picture do not have to meet the legal requirement.[176]

High levels of X-ray emissions will only occur if there is a serious fault in the machine. There are some types of malfunction in the high voltage power supply circuitry that can affect the anode voltage to the VDU to such an extent that the risk of higher radiation doses would be increased dramatically. In some of the older types of VDU with valve rectifiers, the deterioration of the rectifier could, under some circumstances, result in higher radiation emission levels from the VDU. If and when there is a problem from these sources it would be obvious to the operator, because the image on the screen would distort and eventually collapse. Therefore any distortion of the screen image should signal warning, the machine must be turned off and a service engineer called.

Alternatively, you could relieve your frustration and do what the Americans call 'electrobashing', throw the VDU through the window or smash it on a scrap heap. This *clearly* signals the time to buy a new VDU!

No room for complacency

Repeatedly, with the passing of time, new scientific evidence has been produced which reveals that safety standards which had been considered to be safe have been found not to be so after it has been discovered that many people have suffered damaging effects to their health. Accepted safety standards for X-ray emissions have been and still are frequently questioned, reviewed and reduced to lower safer levels, as shown on page 81.

Concern was expressed by Dr C.R. Hirning and Dr J.H. Aitken. According to their calculations, if female operators were exposed to the regulatory limit of 0.5 mR/hr the breasts could receive an annual X-ray dose of 85 mR/yr which is larger than the dose delivered in a mammography procedure. Similarly the annual dose to the thyroid gland could be 190 mR/yr. The authors write, 'While it is true that neither of these hypothetical doses exceeds the current recommended dose limits for individual members of the public (0.5 rem/year) the large and growing number of VDU users could result in substantial collective doses if their units were emitting X-rays at levels close to the limit.'[76]

You can reassure yourself

Reputable manufacturers will provide details of radiation emission levels on all their VDUs (including yours) on request. Ask your employer or school to get the information for you.

If X-ray emissions were a problem for the health of VDU operators, there would have been a greater incidence of ill health than there already is, with additional symptoms which have not been detected.

There have been a number of tests which demonstrated that some rogue VDUs suffering from manufacturing defects have emitted X-rays far above the accepted safety standards (and many more are very close). I have given details of some of these earlier (see page 81). Nonetheless the screens and performance of those VDUs would have made it obvious to the operator that there was something seriously wrong and work would not have been able to continue on them for very long before the entire system crashed.

What you can do

1 Ask employers and schools to provide information from the manufacturer on the X-ray emission levels of the screen, and from the back of the VDU near the flyback transformer.
2 Ensure that thorough six-monthly maintenance checks are carried out.
3 If there is any apparent distortion, flickering, or lack of clarity of the letters on the screen, or if there is any vibration or unusual noise coming out of the unit, then switch it off immediately and don't use it again until a service engineer has checked the machine thoroughly and replaced any imperfect parts.

CHAPTER FOURTEEN
Ionising ultraviolet radiation and ozone

As long ago as 1926, Sir Stewart Duke-Elder reported that ultraviolet had the capability of initiating cataract formations.[83]

Ultraviolet radiation

The natural source of ultraviolet radiation is the sun. Some of the immediate beneficial and adverse effects are familiar to us, varying from gentle warming to browning or burning of the skin to sunstroke. Other adverse health effects of ultraviolet include ageing of the skin, burns on the cornea of the eye, cataracts, conjunctivitis, eye strain and irritation, and skin cancer.

Long-lasting effects may not show up for several years or even decades. In a suntan, the key factor is the length of exposure. For the VDU operator it is the proximity of the source and the length of time and repeated exposures.

There are three different categories of ultraviolet radiation, known as UVA, UVB and UVC. They are identifiable by their wavelengths and are measured in nanometres (nm). Only part of ultraviolet, UVA, falls within the ionising spectrum. UVB and UVC are non-ionising and are discussed in the next chapter.

Because it has been assumed, until recently, that UVA was of little consequence for health, very few detailed investigations have been made specifically in that area. Some current scientific thinking throws doubts on that assumption, suspecting a link between cumulative small doses of exposure to UVA and the growing number of skin cancers and premature ageing of the skin. Jack Shelmerdine at Manchester University told me:

It is now felt that repeated exposure to UVA can cause damage to the skin and eyes. In normal circumstances the body's repair mechanism remedies the damage, but there comes a time when the damage rate exceeds the rate of the body's repair mechanism. Time and repeated exposure are a factor.

He began leading a new intensive research into these cumulative effects in 1988 and the results are awaited. He adds:

Each of these three types of ultraviolet penetrates matter in a different way with the potential for causing biological damage to humans. The more serious hazards to health are considered to come from wavelengths longer than 200 nanometres. Those effects are mainly limited to the eyes and the skin. Long-lasting effects may not show up for several years or even decades.

Safety levels

There are no mandatory safety levels for exposure to ultraviolet radiation. Guidelines supplied by international regulatory agencies suggest a comparison with the standards set for lasers and home television sets of no more than two milliwatts per square centimetre.[82]

In the past, officialdom has recognised that there could be a potential risk to some workers from ultraviolet radiation. Those particularly identified include dentists, hairdressers, laboratory workers, lighting technicians, nurses, physiotherapists, photographic workers and welders. But the official position assumes that there would be no danger to the operators from this source since the average measurements taken from VDUs are usually around five microwatts per square centimetre, which is far below the occupational guidelines. However, many scientists feel that investigations into the VDU operator's special circumstances of working so close to the source during repeated and prolonged periods have not been assessed sufficiently.

The skin

No cases of skin cancer due to occupational exposure have ever been reported – or suspected.

Photosensitisation of the skin to ultraviolet can occur either as a result of genetic causes or contributory chemical causes.

Genetic causes relate to a group of metabolic diseases known as the porphyrias. People who suffer from these produce excess quantities of a sensitising chemical which may result in skin lesions and aversion to light.

Chemical photosensitisation happens in a small proportion of those exposed who develop an allergy from the combination of being exposed to ultraviolet radiation and also to one of a number of chemical agents on the skin or in the atmosphere. The chemical agent could be from a number of sources, such as medicines, cosmetics, industrial chemicals, organic solvents, synthetic dyes in clothing in direct contact with the skin, or even possibly dyes eaten in food. Any one of these combined with ultraviolet can, within an hour or two, irritate or injure the skin and cause a burning sensation, itching or redness – usually in patches.

Medicines swallowed or injected will not produce these symptoms until their chemical reaction has been built up in the skin – that could take several days or weeks. Some drugs are known to be capable of producing temporary photosensitivity, the most common ones being antibiotics and major tranquillisers.

The eyes

The principal effect of ultraviolet damage to the eyes is kerato conjunctivitis, known colloquially as 'arc eye', 'welder's flash' and 'snow blindness'. The symptoms are pain, discomfort similar to a feeling of having grit in the eye and an aversion to bright light. The cornea and conjunctiva become inflamed. The severity depends on the duration, intensity and wavelength of the exposure. The symptoms usually disappear after 36 hours and permanent corneal damage is very rare.

The worst effect on the eye is produced at a wavelength of 270 nanometres.

The more penetrating UVA radiation in the wavelength range of 315 to 400 nanometres has been thought to be absorbed less by the cornea. But it is known that its absorption in the aqueous humour (the liquid filling the cavity between the cornea and the lens) and in the lens itself may produce a transient fluorescent effect which is thought to be harmless but which should serve as a warning of excessive exposure. Absorption of UVA in the lens probably contributes to its progressive yellowing and may be a factor in producing cataracts.[78] Now that there is evidence of cataract formation due to VDU work, some of those case histories are discussed in the next chapter.

Ultraviolet emissions from VDUs produce ozone

Wherever and whenever ultraviolet radiation is produced by high voltages, as it is on our television and VDU screens, a chemical reaction occurs in the surrounding area that creates ozone, which is poisonous to people. Ozone attacks most materials and life forms in its path. Cells on the body surfaces may be damaged if they are overexposed to it.

This added air pollutant in the VDU vicinity is less than would be emitted from a printer or photocopier, but nonetheless adds to ozone emissions already present in many offices and which, in some cases, are ten times over the ozone safety limit.

Screens left on whilst not in use are producing a continuous small amount of ozone which, in buildings without adequate ventilation, will be a contributory factor in the 'sick building syndrome'. Ozone emissions must always be controlled with adequate extraction and ventilation.

Ozone safety levels

The current guidance notes by Britain's Health and Safety Executive were produced in 1983 – before VDUs and laser printers were common on office desks or in schools. There do not appear to be any research figures available for ozone emissions from the VDU screen.

However, new directions were issued in the 1989 Control of Substances Hazardous to Health (COSHH) regulations which mean that companies can be liable for ill health caused by ozone emissions.

Adverse health effects from ozone emissions

The current British safety threshold of 0.1 parts per million is enough to cause
- premature ageing,
- dryness and irritation of the eyes,
- dryness and irritation of the nose,
- dryness and irritation of the throat,

Emissions exceeding 0.5 parts per million can cause
- nausea,
- headaches,
- increased risk of lung infections,

Emissions for two hours at 1.5 parts per million can cause
- coughs,
- excess production of sputum,

At 50 parts per million,
- a 30 minute exposure would result in death.[70]

For more information about ozone and its effects, see Chapter 4.

What you can do

It is not safe to judge the potential danger of ultraviolet radiation by the brightness of the source. Some sources (for example, germicidal lamps) which give off large amounts of ultraviolet radiation give off only a faint visible glow.

1 Keep eyes as far away from the screen as possible. If you need to lean forward to focus on the screen, you need an eye test and new spectacles. Ultraviolet falls off as the square of the distance from the source.
2 The time spent at the screen should be kept to a minimum. Recommended operating times are no more than four hours in one day and no more than one hour without a rest period.
3 Many surfaces, especially those of shiny metal or glossy light-coloured paints, are reflectors of ultraviolet radiation. To reduce the intensity of reflected radiation, desk surfaces and walls should be painted in a dark matt colour.
4 For those few operators who have a sensitive skin, the most effective way to protect the skin is to cover as much of it as possible with clothing. Areas of skin at risk are the backs of the hands, the forearms, face and neck.
5 Pain or discomfort felt to skin or eyes whilst working should act as a signal to switch off the VDU and move away. The effects of repeated exposures may not become apparent for several years.
6 Ensure that the VDU is regularly checked by a competent servicing engineer.
7 If the combination of equipment in the VDU terminal includes intense short wavelength sources, such as laser printers, fluorescent lights and VDU screens, an extraction system should be installed to remove ozone.
8 VDUs must be placed in well ventilated areas.
9 The screen should always be switched off when not in use.
10 Plain glass spectacles with plastic frames afford some protection for the eyes against ultraviolet radiation and reduce the risk of cataracts. But if there is a metal strip within the frame a static charge could build up in the unearthed metal and cause headaches, ear and skin problems. Ferrous metal frames will concentrate the magnetic fields, noble metals are better.

CHAPTER FIFTEEN
Non-ionising ultraviolet, visible light and infrared

A flickering VDU screen can trigger off attacks of photosensitive epilepsy in those who are susceptible.

Viewing letters or pictures produced on the VDU screen is an entirely different concept from looking at the fixed images of motionless words and pictures on a piece of paper or of looking at solid unmoving objects in the surrounding area.

Four major differences must be appreciated. These differences can affect brain patterns, muscles in the neck, arms, back and eyes, and cause headaches, migraine, musculoskeletal problems, eye strain and photosensitive epilepsy.

- The first major difference is that the words and images on the VDU screen are all produced by fluorescence. The degree of brightness and contrast are important factors.

- The second difference is that the letters and images on the screen are never either solid or motionless like the pages of a book or the objects in our natural surroundings, which both our brain and eyes accept as normal. The letters and images on the screen are continually, even if imperceptibly, flickering whilst they are being refreshed.

- The third difference is that three types of radiation are involved in the production of these images; ultraviolet (A, B and C), visible light and infrared (A, B and C).

- The fourth difference is that images from the surrounding area are often reflected in the glass screen, which very often produces glare and can reflect background images. The amount and severity of glare depends on the type and quality of the glass used.

Health effects

Adverse effects of ultraviolet B and C are redness and premature ageing of the skin, premature yellowing of the lens of the eye, cataracts and skin cancers.

Visible and infrared A radiations (with wavelengths between 400 and 700 nanometres) are refracted at the cornea of the eye and brought to a focus on the retina. The retinal and lenticular tissues are most at risk.

Photochemical hazards, which are known to exist with the blue light in the spectrum, and thermal hazards (heating of skin and eyes), are connected to red light and infrared A. They can cause burns on the retina. Chronic effects are cataracts.

Infrared B and C radiations (with wavelengths longer than 1400 nanometres) are quickly absorbed by surface body tissue. Skin and eye burns leading to cataracts have been attributed to these wavebands.[90]

Safety levels

The recommended safety limits are covered under British Safety Standard BS 4830, and proposals by the American Conference of Governmental Industrial Hygienists.[84]

These radiation emissions from the VDU are usually found to be in the region of 1 milliwatt per square centimetre, which is well below the safety levels of 10 milliwatts per square centimetre.[85, 89, 90]

Photosensitive epilepsy

The VDU's method and frequency of transmitting light is basically incompatible with the natural human visual capacity and brain wave patterns. The adverse health effects would depend on the individual operator's physical weaknesses or susceptibility.

An example most of us are familiar with is the extreme condition of fluorescent, pulsating, flickering lights used to spectacular effect in discos and night clubs. They heighten hyperactivity by affecting the brain wave patterns. Whilst this has no long-term adverse effects on most people it does trigger off headaches, dizziness, nausea, epileptic fits, convulsions and heart attacks in those prone to such adverse physical symptoms. In many countries these lights have now been banned.

Whilst the effects from the VDU are not quite so dramatic, nonetheless its flickering screen can be responsible for most of the complaints above and trigger off attacks of photosensitive epilepsy in some people.

Particularly at risk of photosensitive epilepsy are school children between the ages of 10 and 18. The classroom VDU or home computer could cause the first or subsequent attacks. Most of those people who are susceptible will have suffered their first attack before they are 21 and will know to avoid both TV and VDU screens – and flickering light in discos and night clubs.

Medical assessments of the numbers of children likely to suffer photosensitive epilepsy vary between five and twenty out of every 100,000.[86,90]

The flash frequencies produced by the VDU can induce convulsions in susceptible people because they interfere with the natural brainwave patterns. It was assumed that convulsions or epileptic attacks would only happen with frequencies between 10 and 25 Hz but recent studies show that they can be produced between 10 and 43 Hz.[87]

What you can do

1 *Good contrast and sharp focus*. Operators must not only be able to control the contrast and brightness of the images on the screen to suit their individual eyesight but must also remember to perform regular checks

each time the VDU is switched on – and repeatedly throughout the day as lighting conditions change. An imperfectly illuminated screen can easily lead to avoidable stress, eye strain, headaches and even migraine. If the body is badly positioned to compensate, that can lead to an assortment of musculoskeletal disorders which are very often wrongly attributed to office furniture or even to radiation.

It is an understandable operator error because regrettably most computer manuals fail to give adequate instructions how to check and set the brightness and contrast controls for the screen, and far too many give none at all. Frequently the only clues are the symbols on the two control knobs which are usually situated on the VDU casing at the bottom right-hand corner of the screen (others are away from the screen on the side of the VDU casing).

The *contrast* control is usually represented by a circle with one half white and the other half painted black. The *brightness* control also has a circle painted on it with little white dashes coming off around the outside – this is supposed to represent the sun.

Here's how to understand and set the screen to suit your individual eyesight; type a couple of paragraphs and then perform the experiments below:

(a) Turn both brightness and contrast knobs as far to the left as possible so that the screen looks blank.

(b) Slowly turn the contrast control to the right until the letters on the screen become easy to read. As soon as that point is reached you have a screen set for your eyesight. Do not be tempted to make the screen or letters brighter than is necessary.

(c) Sometimes, either because of your eyesight, or ambient lighting in the background, or because of the design of the VDU, you will still not be able to see the letters clearly when the contrast knob is turned as far as possible to the right. In this case slowly turn the brightness control to the right until the letters are in sharp focus and clear enough to be read. Do not intensify the brightness beyond this stage or the letters will begin to fuzz or broaden.

(d) Finally, to become more familiar with the differences in contrast and brightness, perform a few experiments. Turn both knobs to the right to their maximum; you will see the brightness of the letters intensify until they fluoresce, broaden and fuzz. The background colour of the screen will also intensify (for example, what appeared to be a black screen can become quite green, or orange, depending on the chosen background colour). If you then slowly begin to turn the contrast knob back to the left you will notice double and ghosted images along with the trail of the electron beam. All traces of these exaggerated factors must be totally eliminated when working. Even so, you will not be able to avoid the ghosted images on your screen when you scan through a document with the cursor.

Note: because of the difference in individual eyesight it is never a good idea for groups of people, particularly children, to gather around and view one screen together – yet this is a common occurrence. The VDU screen is not a substitute for a blackboard. One screen equates to one person viewing.

2 Because of competitive pricing policies some manufacturers use inferior glass in their screens which results in increased problems with glare and reflections.

The problems of reflections from the surroundings and inappropriate lighting are dealt with in Chapters 23 and 25.

3 A detachable anti-glare screen placed over the VDU screen will reduce or eliminate glare and reflections. It is attached to the VDU casing with adhesive velcro strips. Models should be chosen that are easily removable for daily cleaning with anti-static solutions. In order of efficiency and price, these screens are variously constructed out of (a) polarised glass, (b) tinted glass, or (c) a fine black mesh fabric. They will not afford any protection from either radiation or static – no matter what the manufacturer claims!

4 Antistatic screens look similar to anti-glare screens and will eliminate glare in the same way. The difference is that the mesh screens are made out of a fine carbonised fibre, and most will lose their protective qualities after a short time. All of the antistatic screens have a lead attached to the frame which must be earthed. Details of the alternative ways to do this can be found in the checklist at the end of Chapter 17. The screens must be regularly cleaned with antistatic cleaning solutions. Some manufacturers make claims that these screens will also protect you from radiation emitted by the VDU – that is blatantly untrue.

5 Whilst both types of screen in (3) and (4) above eliminate glare and reflections, they can considerably intensify the flicker and stroboscopic effects of the fluorescent images on inferior VDU screens. That is good because it would alert you to the fact that something is wrong and that you should cease using the VDU.

6 The VDU must be placed on a tilt and swivel stand so that adjustments for personal viewing and to avoid background reflections can more easily be controlled. Part 4 deals with the complexity of creating a safe working environment and the diversity of environmental requirements.

CHAPTER SIXTEEN
Microwaves, radio frequencies, VLF and ELF

These are the most likely sources to cause the majority of miscarriages, birth deformities, reproductive problems, RSI – and several other types of VDU-terminal sickness.

It is most certainly not uncommon for the measurements of electromagnetic radiation around the screen and the casing of the VDU to be far above recommended safety limits. It is assumed that, at the position of the operator, the electromagnetic radiation will have lost sufficient power to cause harmful effects.

Not so good if you are short-sighted and sit with your head close to the screen, or lean your head forward to the desk to read a document. And what about those fingers on the keyboard? Is this why competent typists who suffered no ills on the typewriter have suddenly developed repetitive strain injury (RSI) – because constant repetitive exposure to damaging electromagnetic radiation on the hands can both damage tendons and nerve endings and hinder the natural repair mechanisms? Fingers close to the VDU screen can be exposed to an electromagnetic field of 40,000 volts.

If radiation is responsible for the innumerable clusters of miscarriages and other reproductive problems, this is the most likely source to cause those problems – and several other types of reported VDU terminal sickness.

The effect of these sources of electromagnetic radiation on children whose bodies are still growing is different, and possibly far more serious, from that on adults. The shape, size and angle of the body to the source emitting the radiation are all relevant (shown in Fig 11.4). So too, in the case of the VDU operator, is the conductivity of the floor covering, furnishings and general surroundings.

Many regulatory agencies are still assuming – or hoping – that operators' health would not be at risk from electromagnetic radiation, basing their conclusions on empirical, mathematical and theoretical assumptions. Increasingly, medical and scientific research is demonstrating that these assumptions are hopelessly inaccurate in practice – in the real world, with live human beings.

Empirical assumptions

Until quite recently it has been assumed that if there was no noticeable warming of the body's tissues, then no biological damage would result. Yet already the work of numerous scientists has shown that biological damage to humans can and does occur, without any noticeable heating. We also know that there are different absorption characteristics for small children compared to adults because their growing bodies are still in the developmental stage. Depending on individual physical characteristics some people would be more susceptible to damage. And some parts of the body, like the eyes, hands and gonads, will be more adversely affected. A great deal more research is now being conducted into the effects of the lower frequencies. But research is still very limited, so that a true assessment of the actual damaging effects relating to humans – rather than theoretical estimates of injury – are not conclusively available yet.[104] In particular, information and research on the biological effects of the frequency ranges 15 to 125 kHz are seriously lacking.

When official bodies and manufacturers protest that X-rays from VDUs are not responsible for health problems, and continually make comparisons with the hair dryer and the television,[92-96] that would appear to be a deliberate ploy – to use people's lack of familiarity with radiation in order to direct their attention away from the microwave and radio frequency sources of radiation, knowing, as they must, that when allowances are made for the normal viewing distances from the VDU screen the magnetic fields are 50 to 100 times stronger than during normal television viewing.[94, 96]

Meanwhile the public relations literature from the United Kingdom Atomic Energy Authority assures us that we need not fear any personal harm from radiation from nuclear power stations, pointing out that radiation in the environment from power stations is far less than that which is there from our television sets.[175] And now the additional radiation from millions of VDUs!

Safety levels

There is a problem in accurately measuring many of these emissions because in some areas, particularly some of the lower frequencies, there is a lack of measuring equipment capable of giving accurate readings.

Exposure to microwaves and radio frequency radiation has an additive and cumulative effect.

Safety recommendations to manufacturers in Britain, most of Europe, the USA and Canada are to keep these emissions ALARP – as low as reasonably practicable – or ALARA – as low as reasonably achievable. Neither of these provides a guarantee of safety to the public.

There are no mandatory safety levels.

There are recommended safety levels documented from many different international regulatory agencies which show that there is a wide variety of opinion about just what levels are considered to be safe. In Britain the Medical Research Council and the National Radiological Protection Board (NRPB) have both made recommendations for the protection of the general public.

- The safe exposure level recommended by the NRPB for the frequency range 30 to 30,000 MHz is 10 mW/cm² or, 1mW hour/cm², during any one hour period.
  This is less restrictive than the American National Standards Institute in the VHF and UHF bands (100 MHz to 1.5 GHz). The NRPB did not include considerations relevant to small children which the other two do.[133] Safety levels in eastern European countries are about a factor of ten lower.[134] The West German limits are generally higher.[135]
- There are no recommended safety levels for frequencies up to 30 MHz. It has been assumed that no damage would result from exposure to these frequencies but progressively scientific papers are showing that these

frequencies are capable of producing a multiplicity of adverse health effects. Pulse repetition rates of approximately 8 to 25 Hz are associated with cellular and neurological processes.

- There are no recommended or adopted safety levels that apply to the particular circumstances of the VDU operator who is exposed to several different types of ionising and non-ionising electromagnetic radiation simultaneously.[103]
- In the Soviet Union, where much more research has been done on the 'non-thermal' effects of radio-frequency radiation than in the West, standards are usually at least 100 times more strict than in the West. For microwave radiation Soviet standards are 1,000 times more strict than in many Western countries; only 10 μW/cm^2 are allowed in the USSR. In Canada the permissible level is 1,000 μW/cm^2, whilst in the USA the permissible level is 10,000 μW/cm^2.[131]
- Whilst scientists are not in agreement, the National Institute of Occupational Safety and Health believes there is sufficient evidence of harmful effects to cause concern about human exposures.[132] Further comprehensive investigations are required.

Enforcement of recommended safety standards

The UK Health and Safety Executive (HSE) are responsible for ensuring that there is no danger to the health of workers. Their telephone number and address can be found in your local telephone directory.

At the end of 1990 Nigel Watson from the HSE told me that they did not have the equipment available to conduct tests for radiation but if they felt there was a problem they would call in outside agencies to check the matter out.

Earlier I had spoken to Roger Blakewell from the National Radiological Protection Board who advised me that comprehensive testing of a VDU could be performed by them. But, he warned, such testing would be extremely expensive; the cost of the equipment required to carry out these tests was well in excess of £100,000, testing could take at least a whole day, and they would have to charge for the time of the investigator(s) travelling to the site, performing the work and compiling the report.

He told me that one firm has requested testing of 900 VDUs on their premises but that the NRPB did not have the facilities, staff or equipment to test on such a large scale.

There are only a few companies and consultancies who can perform rigorous testing of VDU terminals.

Adverse health effects from microwaves and radio frequencies

Long ago the USSR and Czechoslovakia conducted full-scale investigations into the health of thousands of people who had been exposed to radio frequency and microwave radiation. Unlike the Western countries, they know that it is irrelevant that these radiations do not have a thermal effect (a noticeable warming of the skin or tissues); they found that they could penetrate right through the human body causing electrical, non-thermal effects which were capable of long-term injury and irreversible damage.

Research findings

Full-scale investigations into the health of thousands of workers exposed to microwaves and radio frequencies show that exposure to microwaves and radio frequencies cause:

- Changes in the brain and central nervous system[111, 112, 121, 127]
- Effects on the eyes, including cataracts[127]
- Changes in the chemistry of the blood and circulatory systems[121]
- Cardiovascular problems (heart and blood vessels)[115, 116]
- Metabolic changes in tissues[115, 116]
- Conditioned reflex behaviour[121, 122]
- Cancer[117-119]
- Leukaemia[119]
- Disruption of cells[117-119]
- Changes in the immunological system (resistance to disease)[115, 116, 121, 124]
- Adverse effects in male reproduction system resulting in
  - reduced sperm count[105, 108, 109, 114]
  - reduced or cessation of ability to have an erection or to ejaculate[108]
  - birth deformities and still-births[105, 108, 109, 128, 130]
  - decrease in libido (sexual drive)[108, 121, 123]
- Adverse effects in female reproduction system which result in
  - disruption of the menstrual cycle[105, 121, 123, 126]
  - adverse reproduction and development of offspring[105, 126, 127]
  - miscarriages[105, 113, 126]
  - birth deformities and still-births[105, 106, 108, 113, 126, 127, 130]
  - decrease in sexual drive[121, 123]

Because very few research programmes relate specifically to VDU operators we look for warning signs in other sectors where investigations have taken place, in other industries and to the results of laboratory tests on animals.

Reproductive problems

1 Women in eastern Europe and the Soviet Union exposed to electromagnetic energy at frequencies in the microwave and radio frequency ranges developed a variety of reproductive and developmental effects. They include changes to menstrual patterns, increased incidence of miscarriage, and decreased lactation in nursing mothers. Retarded foetal development and increased congenital anomalies have been noted among exposed offspring.[105, 126]

2 In Czechoslovakia women of childbearing age have been prohibited from working with radio frequency radiation because of reported changes in menstrual patterns, increased miscarriages and birth defects.

3 The USSR and other eastern European countries prohibited pregnant women from working in areas where microwave levels exceed 10 μW/cm².

4 Exposure of rats to radio frequency energy resulted in numerous foetal malformations including abnormalities of the central nervous system, eye deformities, cleft palate, and deformation of the tail.[127]

5 A Polish study showed that at 10 mW/cm² microwaves caused a large proportion of still-births and deformities at birth in laboratory animals.[106]

6 Workmen exposed to non-ionising electromagnetic energy developed changes in their production of spermatozoa (spermatogenesis) in the testicles.[109] Two additional investigations on male animals reported reproductive effects including testicular damage, debilitated or stillborn offspring and changes in spermatogenesis.[105, 128]

7 A Romanian study of 31 male technicians who had been exposed to microwaves found significantly reduced sperm counts and sperm mobility and an increased proportion of abnormal sperm compared to an unexposed group. Seventy per cent of the technicians showed decreases in libido and problems with erection, ejaculation and orgasm.[108]

8 Children of American military personnel who worked with assorted mechanisms that emitted microwaves demonstrated a significantly higher rate of deformities than those in other sectors of the population.[130]

9 Exposure of pregnant animals to microwaves of 500 μW/cm² resulted in a sevenfold increase in post-natal mortality among the offspring. The survivors had birth weights considerably lower than the norm.[113]

10 The US National Center for Devices for Radiological Health reported that low-level microwave and radio frequency radiation can damage chromosomes. Mice exposed to a level only one eighth of the current exposure standard suffered from a hundredfold increase in defects of sperm chromosomes.[114]

Central nervous system and brain

11 In 1977 Dodge and Glaser found that changes in brain wave patterns could be caused by microwave or radio frequency radiation with power densities of 20 μW/cm².[111]

12 Soviet scientist Dr M.G. Shandala found a 25% decrease in cholinesterase, a substance necessary for nerve cell functioning, in the brains of rats exposed to frequencies of 70 MHz, 155 MHz and 195 MHz at a field intensity of 20 V/m.[112]

Metabolic systems

13 Exposures to microwave and radio frequencies of only 500 μW/cm² are reported to have caused imbalances in potassium and sodium levels which can cause high blood pressure.[115, 116]

Cancer

14 A five-year study by Dr Arthur Guy showed that exposure to 0.48 mW/cm² of microwave and radio frequency radiation caused a significant increase of malignant tumours in rats.[117]

15 The link between cancer and microwave and radio frequency radiation was discovered after extensive research in Poland at the Centre for Radiology and Radio Protection.[118]

16 Mice exposed for short periods developed leukaemia over three times more frequently than those not exposed.[119]

The eyes

The effects of exposure to microwave and radio frequency radiation can continue for many years because they are additive and cumulative. Cataracts in the eyes have been observed to develop between four and twenty-four years after exposure.

17 Ostberg of Sweden was one of the first to recognise the prominence of asthenopic and neurasthenic signs and symptoms in some VDU operators.[160] At that time (1975) the official conclusion drawn was that the problems were entirely due to the unsuitability (for computer use) of existing designs of office furniture and surroundings. Dr Milton Zaret in New York had suspicions and some evidence that non-ionising radiation might possibly be responsible.[161]

18 In the Soviet Union, Sadcikova (1974) had earlier reported a hundred cases of microwave and radio frequency problems. Some of her cases developed cataracts after exposure to 1 mW/cm².[162]

19 Hirsch and Parker (in 1952),[163] Carpenter and Donaldson (in 1970)[164] and Zaret (1974)[165] had all reported cataracts in men following repeated exposures to non-ionising radiation after exposures of around 1.0 mW/cm².

20 As early as 1926 Sir Stewart Duke-Elder had shown that radiation – from the longest wavelengths generated by oscillations to the shortest wavelengths of ionising radiation – had the ability to initiate cataract formation.[166]

21 Bouchat and Marsol of France reported the case of a radar technician whose eyes were normal when he began work at the age of nineteen. Over the next four years they observed him develop capsular cataracts which were attributed to microwave radiation exposure. By differential diagnosis they ruled out any other known causal factors.[167]

22 A female VDU operator acquired an unilocular incipient cataract in one eye after working with VDUs for eighteen months, a bizarre illness that started with a partial loss of hearing in one ear associated with tinnitus, loss of balance, and a loss of pupillary reactions. Extensive clinical and laboratory testing, including neurological, otological and ophthalmological consultations, failed to find any explanation for any of her symptoms until Dr Milton Zaret found the incipient cataract in her left eye (her right eye also exhibited early signs of non-ionising radiation injury).[168]

23 Over the years Zaret had experience of many hundreds of cases of cataracts and other eye problems that had developed after the workers' eyes had been exposed to very low doses of microwave and radio frequency radiation, so he was not surprised that these problems began to show up in VDU operators. In 1980 Zaret reported eight cases of cataracts following use of VDUs. Since that time a great many more have come to his notice; some, including a famous case involving reporters who operated VDUs at the *New York Times* resulted in litigation. Zaret says that the effects of exposure can continue for many years.

In one of his papers Zaret describes how sometimes what appear to be unrelated symptoms might give the early warning signs. These include:

(a) problems in neurological functions and in special sense organs like the ear.

(b) a partial loss of hearing.

(c) blurred vision.

(d) different colour sense in each eye (anisometachromatopsia).

(e) loss of pupillary reactions.

(f) difficulties with balance (vestibular dysfunction).

(g) eye fatigue and distress because of a muscle imbalance in the two eyes working as a team (asthenopia).

(h) headaches just above the eyes.

(i) nuclear sclerosis (the central portion of the lens becomes opaque, which can lead to an opacity of the entire lens). Nuclear sclerosis can be a sign of premature abnormal ageing – another known effect of radiation.

In 1982, Zaret expressed concern over the recommended safety standards, citing many cases where cataracts and other eye problems have resulted from exposures below the recommended standards. He said that European and American standards were wrong, pointing out that the current permitted exposure level at 10 mW/cm² takes no account of the length of the exposure. He pointed out that for continuing exposure one should be exposed to not more than 1 mW/cm². For one tenth of an hour per hour this could rise to 10 mW/cm².

He also pointed out that the temperature and humidity in the office can confuse the effects of the radiation emissions. He writes:

When there is a rise above 70 degrees F. but below 79 degrees F., there needs to be a reduction in the permissible radiation levels. Ultimately, for a temperature/humidity index over 79 degrees F., only a tenth of 1 mW is permitted. That is 100 µW/cm². However, none of the measuring equipment used in any of the surveys were sensitive to that level, as far as I am aware.

. . . The standards are set for normal healthy adults. With certain sicknesses such as circulatory problems, the radiation levels should be reduced further by a factor of ten . . . Unfortunately the standard setting committees are not the people who will have to apply these standards; instead, people like us will have to. It should be understood that, as a general rule, the more dogmatic and firm people are in their statements about radiation safety, the less they really know about the subject.[168]

General findings

24 Reported observations at relatively low energy levels in laboratory rats or rabbits have included changes in electrical activity in the brain,[121] conditioned reflex behaviour,[121, 122] chemical composition of the blood,[121] the endocrine (hormonal) system,[121, 123] and the immune system.[121, 124].

For the frequencies at which these observations have been made, the rates of energy absorption in humans are much greater than in the laboratory animals,[125] so the effects observed in animals may occur in humans at even lower exposure levels.

25 Dr Karel Marha feels that any change in behaviour patterns such as the onset of weariness, inability to concentrate, sluggishness, headaches, dizziness, mental depression and eye pains,[110] involuntary reactions or muscle contractions[12] should be taken as early warning signs that more serious problems could be imminent. If any of these symptoms occur the VDU operator's health and the emissions in the terminal should be checked.[110]

26 Czechoslovakian scientists report that these types of radiation can interfere with trace metals which might be deposited in the body for medical reasons.[120] Manufacturers of metallic surgical implants, such as copper IUDs used for birth control and pacemakers for the heart, issue similar warnings to those who have them.

Pulsed electromagnetic fields: extremely low frequency (ELF) and very low frequency (VLF) radiation

During the past few years growing suspicions have progressively been backed up by scientific evidence which confirms that the electromagnetic fields of these low frequencies can and do cause observable effects:

- Changes in the heart and the brain.[136]
- Observed changes in human cells exposed to these frequencies could, under certain circumstances, promote cancer.[137]
- Additionally some studies show a large proportion of deformities and mortality in chicken embryos indicating that birth defects and mortality in human offspring might be affected similarly. Later tests conducted in Sweden on cells taken from women also showed the same disruptive effects.[138]
- Changes in the chromosomes could lead to various kinds of diseases.[138]

Sources of ELF and VLF

This type of radiation is an invisible and unwanted side product of the supply of electricity via underground and overhead electric power cables and the network of pylons that spread across the country. Equally most electrical devices emit electric and magnetic fields; for example, fluorescent lighting, navigational equipment, electrical tools, cooking devices, radios, televisions, electric blankets, food mixers, heating pads and VDUs.

The effects to humans of the electromagnetic emissions from these electrical appliances are dependent on the particular characteristics of the electrical appliance used, the distance you are away from it and the length of time that it is used.

Exposure to the electric field can sometimes be felt because it can make skin or hair tingle. The magnetic field cannot be felt and it cannot be avoided – it travels through most materials in its path including humans, animals, plants, roofs, bricks, glass and concrete.

Who is most at risk?

Groups of people who have been exposed to repetitive dosages of the low frequency electromagnetic fields are:

1 Those in electrical occupations, including television and radio service engineers. Reporting on research into old records of people in this occupational group, Dr Samuel Millam, an epidemiologist with the Seattle Department of Health, found earlier and higher death rates amongst this occupational group when compared to the statistics of other sectors of the community. [146-149]

2 People living under or close to electric pylons and overhead cables, and,

3 VDU operators. If you refer back to the end of Chapter 11 you will find how and where ELF and VLF are produced by the VDU.

Safety levels

VLF and ELF emitted by the VDU are well in excess of even the maximum recommended safety levels, but because of the fall of power with distance, they are expected to be below the present recommended safety levels at 'normal' viewing distance. However, we are still in the early days for research into the health risks and safe levels from these pulsed electromagnetic fields. The current safety standards and working practices will most probably be amended repeatedly – just as those have for X-ray exposure.

Research findings

1 Among the first to suspect that weak magnetic fields may have hazardous health effects on people were Wertheimer and Leeper in 1979 and 1982. They found a greater incidence of cancer among people living in higher magnetic fields. [149-151]

2 The earliest tests that demonstrated that miscarriages and birth defects can be caused by magnetic fields like those emitted from the VDU were conducted in Spain in 1982 and 1983 by Delgado et al.[140]

The operator, seated in front of the VDU, is mostly shielded from the electrical component of the varying VLF electromagnetic field. But, the magnetic field cannot be avoided by the VDU operator.

Delgado and his team used chick embryos to try to find the interaction mechanism between magnetic fields and the body's biological system. The results of these tests clearly demonstrated a considerable increase in the number of abnormalities in 48-hour-old chick embryos, resulting in a large proportion of dead or deformed chicks.

Delgado's result revealed an unsuspected curiosity. The chick embryos were damaged or destroyed when they were exposed to 100 Hz magnetic pulses. Oddly, the same effects did not occur at higher (1000 Hz) or lower (10 Hz) frequencies. This demonstrated what is now called a window effect.[140]

Delgado's principle of the 'window effect' demonstrated that less is often more harmful than more, showing that a lower strength of, or frequency of exposure to, magnetic fields can be much more damaging than a higher one. If that really is so then the logical and mathematical assumptions (relied upon by scientists and officialdom) did not reveal the truth about what actually happens to humans exposed to these VLF and ELF electromagnetic fields.

The exposures quoted by Delgado from his experiments are a *thousandfold less than the British safety limit* of 20 teslas recommended by the NRPB!

Delgado's results were so important that they aroused a great deal of controversy. For almost a decade there have been rejections and denunciations of his findings from other scientists and regulatory bodies. The mere mention of his name has frequently brought a derisory snigger from officialdom. A few other groups of 'officially approved' scientists claimed that they tried to repeat Delgado's experiments without success.

In a report in the *British Medical Journal* in October 1985 Dr Lee, Professor of Occupational Health at Manchester University, wrote:

We can only speculate on the relevance of these findings to events inside a uterus within a human body some 30 to 100 cm from a VDU screen. If the concept of a window effect, particularly with regard to field strength, were to be established it would greatly complicate the task of the epidemiologist looking for a conventional 'dose effect' relation.[170]

The safety levels recommended by the NRPB for nuclear magnetic resonance[171] are based on the possibility of the magnetic currents causing depolarisation in nerve and muscle cells rather than on possible adverse effects to the unborn foetus. Nonetheless there is a cautionary note of uncertainty in the NRPB guidelines. These state:

Although there is evidence to suggest that the developing embryo is not sensitive to magnetic fields encountered in nuclear magnetic resonance, clinical

imaging studies (yet to be confirmed) reported changes which could have
*developmental consequences. It was considered prudent therefore, on this
tentative evidence, to* exclude pregnant women during the first trimester
when organ development is taking place in the embryo until more
conclusive evidence is forthcoming. *(My emphasis).*

So far as I am aware, neither the Health and Safety Executive nor the
NRPB have made these doubts known to VDU users, employers or
trade unions.[170]

3 It was not until 1986 that similar results to Delgado's were produced in
two tests by Juutilainen et al. when the abnormality rate in the embryos
reached 56%.[141-143] By 1991 Delgado's results have been replicated by
other groups from different countries.

4 A Polish study in 1986 exposed both male and female rats to the
radiation beneath a black and white television set. The results showed a
number of deformities and a lower litter weight among offspring from
the females who had been exposed. The exposed male rats suffered a
significant reduction of weight in the testicles.[144]

5 Intensive monitoring of the effect that electromagnetic radiation from the
VDU has on women working in the VDU terminal was carried out
within a project by the Central Institute of Labour Safety in Poland.
They concluded that (a) VDUs are the source of low intensity
electromagnetic radiation with a complex nature; (b) the incidence of
miscarriages was higher in VDU operators than in another group of
women who did not work with VDUs; and (c) there is a susceptibility of
the neuroendocrine system to the VDUs' electromagnetic fields. They
recommended not employing pregnant women on VDUs.[145]

6 Until 1988 the possibility of any connection between the numerous
clusters of cancer and childhood leukaemia among those living close to
electric pylons and overhead cables has been vehemently denied by the
electricity supply companies and regulatory bodies. But fears about
possible harmful effects from these low frequency electromagnetic waves
grew with the observance of the increased number of some cancers in
adults, and leukaemia in children, in those communities who lived
under or close to electric pylons and overhead cables.

A great deal of research has particularly been conducted into these
effects in Denver, Colorado, and Middletown, the growing and densely
populated suburb of New York. In England similar worries have centred
on Failsworth near Oldham in Lancashire and Didcot in Oxfordshire.[188]

Complacency of manufacturers and the electrical power companies
was shaken by Dr David Savitz who found that the fears and connections
of health effects from the power supply were not groundless. He
reported that, depending on the demand on the electricity supply, the
fields from ordinary street lines can be similar to those surrounding
pylons.[183, 184] Controlled scientific investigations into these problems are
still being conducted. Already a number of results of investigative
scientific and epidemiological research have been published and we will
look at some of those now.

7 After the Savitz report from America in 1987, followed since then by a considerable number of other international investigations which show the same and additional effects on humans from the magnetic fields, concern has seen to be shown by the Electric Power Research Institute (EPRI) in America which has provided $3.5 million for further research. Similarly in Britain the Central Electricity Generating Board (CEGB) has made a provision of £500,000 for further research. However neither accepts that there is any cause for alarm, simply because it has been shown that these electromagnetic waves can have an effect on the heart and the brain.

The official position is perhaps best summed up by Dr Leonard Sagan of the EPRI who, after receiving the results of these researches, in an interview said, 'There's a mystery, it's curious. But premature to draw conclusions.' Whilst he accepts, from recent research, that there is now scientific and statistical evidence resulting from measured tests on humans that there are detectable changes in the brain, the heart and cells, caused by exposure to magnetic fields, he cannot say whether those changes are harmful. He adds – they might be beneficial! He sees no cause for alarm at this stage.[188]

8 Dr Nancy Wertheimer and Dr Ed Leeper published a paper in the *American Journal of Epidemiology* showing a link between exposure to electricity power lines and leukaemia in children, and an increase in cancer rates among men in occupations with exposures to magnetic fields.[149] A similar later report by Wertheimer and Leeper confirmed similar findings.[150, 151] Dr Ruey Lin of the Maryland Department of Health and Mental Hygiene found that a significantly higher proportion of workers who died of brain tumors had been employed in electrical occupations such as electricians, electric or electronic engineers and service personnel.[156]

9 Conducting extensive research on young adults in his Kansas laboratory, Dr Charles Graham from the Mid West Institute found low frequency magnetic fields interfered with the body in such a way as to cause serious changes in two of the body's fundamental processes – a slowing down of the heart beat and a reduced ability to concentrate.

After repeated testing he consistently found that exposure to the lower frequencies caused a disruption of normal heart and brain patterns whilst exposure to higher frequencies had no effects. Dr Graham concluded that these wavebands do not behave according to preconceived assumptions. Less (lower frequencies) is worse (more harmful).[188]

10 The US Department of Energy and Utilities recently sponsored a $500,000 investigation to be conducted by Australian-born Dr Ross Adey, a professor of medicine in California and also the White House scientific adviser on magnetic fields. Dr Adey has discovered a cancer connection with these lower electromagnetic frequencies in what is now known as the 'whispering cell theory'.

He explains that within the body it is necessary that cells communicate with each other. They do this by passing signals and chemicals from one cell to another. If these signals are interfered with, the cells will behave in a cancerous way. In doing that they will lose their ability to control their own growth and this will lead to the formation of a tumour. He says that electromagnetic fields can aid cancer-promoting substances in producing a condition of disrupted intercellular communication. Either alone, or together with the cancer-promoting substances, they will produce the promotion stage in the behaviour of the cells which is the beginning of the cancer state. He also has evidence that the electromagnetic field may act as a promoter of the cancer chemical. He says that if you put both together, you see much stronger evidence of the joint effects.[188]

11 Earlier work by Dr Ross Adey showed that cells exposed to 15 Hz fields of 0.1 mV/cm resulted in a loss of 90% of calcium ions from body cells. These ions are charged particles that play a vital role in many different parts of cellular processes, including the transmission of nerve impulses. Adey's results have been confirmed by many others who have replicated his investigations.[152-154]

12 Dr Kjell Hansson-Mild, a leading international biophysicist from the University of Umea in Sweden, has found that these lower frequencies cause changes in the frontal nervous system, the heart and the central nervous system. He conducted one of the six worldwide tests that confirmed Delgado's findings that disruption of the chicken embryos would result in deformed or dead chicks. Later experiments by Dr Hansson-Mild showed changes in the chromosomes from women which could lead to different types of diseases.[188]

13 Dr Stefan Nordstrom of the University of Umea in Sweden has reported that children born to men who work in high voltage situations have an increased incidence of congenital malformations. The study also revealed a decrease in male fertility.[155]

14 Scientific studies into the effects of electromagnetic radiation from the lower frequencies in the USSR have shown bone deformities and still-births in animals.[157]

Whilst research into these ELF and VLF fields continues, a man who has probably studied the effects more comprehensively than most – Dr Michael Coleman, a leading epidemiologist from the World Health Organisation – ended a recent interview by saying:

Possibly our physiology may not be well adapted to exposure to such magnetic fields. It is only since the discovery of electricity that these problems have arisen.

Certainly the occurrence of these types of health problem has increased parallel to our increasing consumption of electricity – used for radio, television, VDUs and a host of other electrical equipment. In his recent book, *Electropollution*, Roger Coghill links electromagnetic radiation from such sources to a great many health hazards, including AIDS and the increase in cot deaths. He explains;

In 1920 only about 90 kW/hours of electricity per head of population in Britain was consumed. By 1987 the figure has grown nearly fifty times, each person now consumes a massive 4,400 kW/hours of electricity.[191] *This electric energy is distributed by 14,571 kilometres of mains lines, of which nearly 10,000 kilometres are 400 kV power lines, not used before the early 1960s. In this way we are all bringing electromagnetic fields of a myriad types into our homes, oblivious of the effects they may be having on our brains and our bodies.*[176]

How to protect yourself

1 VDUs with plastic casing do not usually give adequate (if any) protection from these types of radiation. Lining the VDU case with earthed copper foil causes a dramatic decrease in the electromagnetic fields of microwaves and radio frequencies from the back of the VDU near the flyback transformer. Presence or absence of adequate shielding varies with different manufacturers, and with different models from the same manufacturer. Most older models will not have this shielding, whilst newer ones usually do. The price and age of the VDU will be a good indicator.

    If your model has not got sufficient built-in protection then your maintenance or service engineer can supply or make an earthed copper foil shield to fit externally around your individual VDU.

2 Your average exposure to a VDU should not exceed between two and four hours daily, with regular periods spent away from the VDU after each period of one hour.

3 When the VDU is not in use, *switch it off*. Even if you are not actually using the VDU you are exposed to electromagnetic radiation when it is switched on. I know that a common reason for leaving VDUs on all day is that it takes too much time to 'get out of the programme' (switch it off) and to 'boot it up' (switch it back on again). That is an in-built characteristic of the computer system. The priority must be operators' health – not employers' convenience, productivity or profitability. Employers must be made to appreciate this.

4 The Australian Radiation Laboratory found that large increases in radio frequency radiation are proportional to contrast and brightness on the screen. Therefore, adjust the brightness and contrast, if necessary, every time you switch on. (If you are not sure how to do this, see Chapter 15). And, switch the VDU off when not in use.

5 From the end of 1992 in Europe it will be the employer's responsibility to provide regular eye and eyesight tests for employees working with VDU screens.

    Other periodical medical checks will probably become the legal requirement one day. Only if and when that happens on a large scale will VDU operators know (rather than assume or imagine) exactly what effects and changes are taking place in their bodies.

    On the one hand such testing would cost far less than VDU-related health problems do at the present time, because if such tests were seen as preventative medicine, health problems could be dealt with at an early stage, and far more cheaply than at present when each country's health service picks up the full cost of treatment after the full-blown symptoms have appeared. Alternatively, as is now the case with eye tests, the cost could be the responsibility of employers.

Meanwhile you could make arrangements with your doctor to arrange to do the requisite medical checks for you. The tests should include:

(a) an electrocardiograph
(b) blood counts
(c) blood chromosome tests
(d) eye examination for cataract
(e) an EEG (electroencephalographic recording of electrical activity in the brain)
(f) ears and hearing checks.

Some British family doctors have pointed out that, because of new National Health Service contract pressures on their time, they may find it difficult to perform all of these tests for the large numbers of VDU users who should have them. Nonetheless these tests are important for people using VDUs, whether they are performed by their local doctor or whether government bodies arrange for separate occupational health specialists to conduct the tests. That controversy is outside the scope of this book.

Because of the increase in industrial and occupational health problems, the time is certainly fast approaching when all family doctor practices will need to use the expertise of a doctor who can not only recognise and treat these new ills, but also provide regular preventative advice and services.

6 A spiderwort plant (Tradescantia) on your desk might provide an early warning of mutagenic and carcinogenic danger. This little plant changes flower colour when mutations occur. It is very sensitive to radiation and (if you have a microscope) can be used to measure radiation levels in an office.[1]

7 The Institut de Recherches en Géobiologie at Chardonne in Switzerland have researched the effects of radiation on an assortment of trees, shrubs and plants. They claim that *Cereus peruvianus*, a small cactus (40 cm high) placed on the work-top near the VDU screen will absorb some of the radiation from the electromagnetic field. High-flyers working on the money-markets on Wall Street who used to suffer repetitive headaches and tiredness no longer have these problems since putting these cacti on and around their work-tops.

8 *Know who to complain to if you feel there is a radiation problem with your VDU*

   (a) A good servicing engineer from your supplier will be able to either check and remedy all of the problems – or advise that the machine should be scrapped. Stand by and watch that the job is done thoroughly and for your records make a note of the instruments used to check the exact radiation levels at each frequency and the exact measures recorded from your VDU.

   (b) In the UK, contact the Health and Safety Executive (whose telephone number is in your local directory). In other countries, contact the appropriate health regulatory body.

Survive with a little knowledge and a big sense of humour

Regrettably – even today – you will often meet with a mixture of ignorance, incompetence and a subjective miserly bias from some less reputable suppliers and manufacturers. By the time you have finished reading the book, and tucked it away for reference in a handy drawer next to the VDU, you will have all the information you need to sort the good guys out from the bad. And to put the condescending arrogant ones in their place.

Below are a few typical responses friends have had from their caring suppliers who are charging a fortune for a maintenance contract:

1 Most people who use a VDU are familiar with this scene; there you are with an important piece of work that is needed most urgently, and time is running out. *Something* goes wrong with the VDU.

Stressed, harassed and worried about radiation from the malfunctioning VDU, you ring the help-line, and it rings, and it rings.

The phone is eventually answered and a sweet relaxed voice asks you to hold the line for a moment! Valuable minutes are passing, you can feel stress and tension building up inside your body, as you know that not only are the minutes rushing by but you might also have lost some of the work from the past few hours. You have probably got a headache already.

Then your ears are assaulted by slow, happy, repetitively rhythmic, prickly music, from an old-fashioned music-box. Even worse, you might get 'Greensleeves' or 'Who is Sylvia?'!

2 The managing director of one very large British computer supply company told me;

'We don't have any facilities to test radiation levels. The administrative controls and instrumentation required would be far too operationally and financially burdensome.'!

3 Another regrettable response I got when I asked another national supplier to visit my VDU and check it for radiation was: 'If there is something wrong the VDU will crash and then we will come out and fix it.'

I persisted: 'If someone used a VDU for a few years, is it not possible that radiation could pose a little problem without the VDU crashing?'

'No. That's impossible,' he said, 'they all crash two or three times a year and any problems would be spotted then because there would be a faulty part and we would notice it and put it right.'

I pointed out: 'I have used my VDU for more than five years and it has never crashed. But, fresh flowers placed near it die within a day whilst other flowers in another room live for a week or more.'

'You must be a very careful owner and have a very good PC,' he said.

'What about zapping my roses and possible radiation?' I asked. 'Can you test the radiations?'

'Well, your flowers are quite a mystery,' he said. 'Perhaps you should contact a florist. We can't help with your flowers or test radiation. We are here to look after computers and get them going again when they crash.'!

4 Fay Vernon, an author and friend, tells me that she telephoned her company's VDU supplier and said that she thought there were troubles with her flyback transformer.

They tried to put her off and make her feel ridiculous. They condescendingly explained: 'VDU's don't have any transformers in them – they all work off electronic circuit boards.'

'Yes, I know about the circuit boards,' she said, 'but there is something wrong with my VDU and I think it's the flyback transformer, and I must say, I am a bit worried about radiation.'

'I've tried to explain, there aren't any transformers inside VDU's,' he insisted, and, he patiently explained, 'flies can't get inside the casing, it's all sealed – unless you've been tampering with it. And, all these tales about radiation are propaganda by the unions and the press. There is *no radiation* in a VDU. Now would you like me to send somebody round to look at your VDU?'

'No, thank you.' She found another servicing company to conduct the necessary checks and repairs, vowing to be much more careful about the choice of a future supplier!

5 Journalists tell me of a simple warning test that they use to check for the presence of hazardous radio frequencies. They tune a transistor radio to a VHF station and hold it close to the VDUs. As you move around each VDU you can tell where the emissions are strongest by listening to the interference on the sound. Then howl for protection.

6 Adding a little mystique, Jake Fox claims that if you put a large quartz crystal on top of the VDU it will absorb some of the electric field, ions and electrons. The crystal must be thoroughly washed once or twice daily in plenty of fresh running cold water to remain effective.

A British firm based in Leeds (Ordosan Ltd) sells crystals and claims in its literature, 'When the cosmoton is worn on the chest or placed on the television or VDU screen, it helps by protecting people in tolerating the radiation far better without ill-effect'.

When we put a large clean crystal on top of the VDU, readings of the radiation emissions showed a considerable reduction of radio frequencies and positive ions in the air in front of the screen. I can't find out why this happens, but it was pointed out to me that the early radio sets used crystals to receive the radio frequencies which were then amplified.

CHAPTER SEVENTEEN
Static

A build-up of static can cause random hissing, crackling and other disturbances on telephones, radios and televisions. It can also distort data inside computers and even cause them to break down completely. Something that can have such a catastrophic effect on electronic equipment can also cause damage to the human body. Dr Leslie Hawkins from Surrey University says: 'The positive charge on the outside of the VDU screen can be 50,000 volts positive.'

Static electricity does not travel in wave-like motions along a current like other types of radiation. Nor does it radiate energy. Nonetheless it is capable of giving you an electric shock and interfering with your health and well-being in complex ways.

Contrary to the outdated assumptions and assurances of manufacturers and official regulatory bodies – on which present health and safety guidelines are based – there is mounting scientific evidence that non-ionising pulsed electromagnetic static fields can, and do, cause biological damage to humans. Their interaction with the organisms of the body is more complex than other types of radiation. Static has been found to cause an assortment of health problems, some for reasons which are scientifically acknowledged but not entirely understood, but all of which are dependent on the duration of exposure and the intensity of the field to which the operator is exposed.

Ions and static

We cannot consider static – particularly in the VDU environment – without understanding a little about the presence of both negative and positively charged ions in the surrounding atmosphere and their interaction.

Ions can exist in the atmosphere if an electron is added to or removed from a gas molecule. The addition of an electron gives a negative ion, the removal gives a positive ion.

High charges of static affect the balance of these ions by destroying the negative ions and leaving the surrounding air with too many positive ones.

Health problems associated with static build-up or with the depletion of negative ions include:

- Biological reaction in adrenals, eyes, heart, kidneys, liver, sinuses and in the white blood cells.
- Problems with the reproductive systems. In women these include ovarian malfunction, loss of libido, haemorrhage, hormonal imbalances, miscarriages, still-births and deformed foetus. In men; reduced weight of testicles, reduced fertility and virility.

113

- Swelling and tingling of the ankles, feet, fingers, wrists and hands; burning sensations in the fingers, wrists and feet.
- Damage to nerve endings in the fingers (scalloped nerve endings).
- Aching joints.
- Muscular function effects in back, neck, arms, hands, fingers and legs.
- Skin problems including sweating, itching, eczema, spots, rashes, dryness and premature ageing.
- Difficulty in breathing, bronchial diseases and asthma.
- Bitter taste in the mouth and tooth pains.
- Blurred vision, dry and itching eyes and conjunctivitis.
- Damaged brain tissues.
- Chest pains.
- Lethargy, dizziness, tension, depression, anxiety, headaches and migraines, tiredness and insomnia.
- Lowered resistance to disease.
- Impaired nerve impulses.
- Thrombosis.
- Malfunction of the thyroid gland.
- Alterations in heart-beat patterns and blood circulation.

Where the static comes from

The static emitted from the VDU originates from the electrical power used to operate the device and also from the electron beam which is directed on to the screen. Ideally the screen should serve as a shield and stop the residual static from leaving the VDU casing. However, because of the limited absorption ability of the glass, the screen provides imperfect shielding.[7] Pulsed static coming from the flyback transformer (which is usually located at the back corner of the terminal) has been found to be even stronger. These will affect persons sitting behind the VDU. A person sitting 100 cm from the rear corner will experience the same field as a person sitting in front of the VDU just 30 cm from the screen. Unless it is redirected (earthed), this electromagnetic static charge will accumulate in and around the operator's body.

The strength of this electrostatic charge can vary considerably depending upon the individual VDU's characteristics,[15] the brightness of the display, the number of characters on the screen at any one time and the rate at which the writing beam scans the screen.[3]

In one test measurements of static close to the screen were recorded to vary on different machines between −150 V/m and +1500 V/m.[4] On many other occasions they have been measured as high as 30 kV/m. The 'average' static field between a VDU and its operator is estimated at +2,500 V/m, although tests have shown that between +10,000 and +50,000 volts is not unusual.

Dr Leslie Hawkins from Surrey University told me:

The positive charge on the outside of the VDU screen can be 50,000 volts positive. There is no current involved so the operator won't get a shock. But, the static field does act as a particle expiator which can accelerate allergic reactions on the skin. The nose, cheek bones, and backs of hands are most likely to be afflicted. In the summer months when less and lighter clothing is worn and more skin is exposed, the problems extend to the shoulders, arms, neck and the chest.

Invisible signs of the presence of static

A build-up of static electricity can make its presence noticed by causing random hissing, crackling and other disturbances on telephones, radios and televisions. It can distort data within the computer and even cause it to break down completely. It doesn't take a great deal of imagination to realise that it is unlikely that operators' health will benefit or remain unaltered by something that can have such a catastrophic effect on electronic components.

Most of us have experienced sensations or little electric shocks caused by static electricity. Here are a few of the common occurrences;

- If we put our fingertips on the television screen whilst it is switched on we feel tingling sensations caused by the electrostatic building up on the outside of the screen.
- If we touch a metal object whilst we are on a synthetic carpet, that can generate quite a sharp electric shock to the hand and arm. A person walking across a synthetic carpet may charge himself or herself to more than 10,000 volts.
- Girls often experience electric shocks – and sometimes see sparks fly – when they touch a clinging petticoat made from a synthetic fabric, or some other garment whose fabric is wholly or partly made from synthetic fibres.
- There is the really freaky hair-raising effect caused by brushing fine hair with a nylon hair brush. The static generated makes the individual hairs defy gravity, float skyward and stand on end – until the static electricity is discharged.
- In some circumstances the discharge of static will produce a spark and in the presence of flammable gases, as in an operating theatre or a coal mine, or of certain dusts, such as wheat or aluminium, there may be an explosion.[32]
- Children have fun with the old party trick of rubbing a blown-up balloon on their chest: then, putting the balloon on a wall where it stays put – stuck up there on the wall – as if by magic.

Natural environmental levels of static

Naturally occurring static is in the air around us. At ground level, during fair weather, it measures about 130 to 150 V/m. Weather conditions, altitude, humidity and pollution can cause this measurement to vary. Static fields of 3,000 V/m are often produced before and during thunderstorms,[5] causing changes in the negative and positive ions in the air.

Natural environmental levels of ions

Research shows that up to three-quarters of the population are physically or mentally affected by an imbalance in negative and positive ions. An atmosphere charged with too many positive ions will induce in operators depressive mood swings and headaches of varying severity, including migraines.[177, 178]

After a thunderstorm the air feels fresher and people feel more exhilarated because the dry air before the storm was charged with positive ions. After the storm the air has a much higher humidity level and a more healthy negative ion balance has been restored. That is why many people prefer to spend hot sunny days near a waterfall, the sea or a swimming pool because in these locations they feel comfortable and far more energetic than they do in a hot, dry climate. The reason they prefer a location near water is because the air is charged with more negative ions, the humidity is higher and the detrimental effects of static and an excess of positive ions have been reduced.

The Department of Human Biology and Health at Surrey University took measurements of the air in various locations familiar to us all. Table 17.1 shows their findings. They demonstrate that our cities in general – and particularly modern air-conditioned office blocks equipped with computers, VDUs and a general assortment of hi-tech equipment – are the most unhealthy places to live or to work. 'Hi-tech electronic smog' is the term used in the USA to describe this new man-made environment.

Table 17.1 Measurements of ion in the air.[41]

	Number of ions per cc of air	
	positive	*negative*
Outdoors: pollution-free country air	1,200	1,000
lightly polluted town air	800	700
city air	500	300
Indoors: rural house no air conditioning	1,000	800
rural office with air conditioning	150	100
city office with air conditioning	100	50

Personal levels of static

Our bodies contain static which gives measurable readings varying between −10 Kv to +10 Kv.

Everyone's body generates static electricity, in some people more than others. The amount of personal static can vary according to the fabrics in our clothes, the floor surfaces we are standing or walking on and the surrounding air.

Some people, particularly those who have a dry skin, are more susceptible to adverse effects from static because dry skin holds and builds up the electric charge.

Although we are usually unaware of it we are constantly receiving and discharging small amounts of static. As we lift one foot from the floor an electrostatic charge is generated from the contact of the foot with the ground. The body's electrostatic charge usually leaks back to earth through the other foot when it is placed on the ground. During this process the static energy stored within the body is quite small but it is still sufficient to create a spark and – in the appropriate circumstances – an explosion.[32]

Alternatively, if the density of static is lowered by spreading the area of contact, such as by firmly grasping a metal key, then the body's personal static can be discharged quite dramatically, as in some of the examples given earlier.

If the charge slowly dissipates over a wide area, as through the soles of the feet, nothing at all is felt. This happens, for example, if the person walks on to a conducting surface or takes off his or her shoes. However if the feet are on a surface which will not allow the charge to be discharged, there will be a greater build-up of a higher voltage within the body which can give rise to shocks.

Natural fibres are conductive because they have a water content which means that they remove the static charges which are attracted to them. Therefore VDU operators wearing only natural fibres, whose shoes have leather uppers and soles, and who work or walk on wool carpets, will not suffer from the static-related problems as much as a counterpart wearing some or all synthetic fibres in their under and over layers of clothing and working or walking on a synthetic or partly synthetic floor covering.

We already know that the officially estimated 'average' static field between a VDU and its operator is 2,500 V/m, but that it has been recorded to be as high as 50,000 V/m in some cases. This is an areas where scientists disagree with each other and produce dramatically different measurements. Careful examination of the results demonstrates that the variance results from the different emissions of individual VDUs. It is dependent on the quality of components used in the manufacturing process, the installation and the surroundings in which the VDU is working.

A Norwegian researcher at the Christian Michaelson Institute in Bergen found that the VDU operator developed a negative charge of 2,200 volts when her VDU had a positive 12,000 volt charge on the screen. He explains that 'Negative ions are attracted to the screen and positive ions and particles in the air are repelled from the screen to the operator's face, resulting in negative ion depletion.'[9]

Discharging static

Floor coverings made wholly or partly from synthetic materials do not allow the build-up of static, either on the VDU or on the human body, to discharge itself through the floor. Therefore, unless the floor covering is made entirely from natural fibres, there is an additional build-up of static electricity which will discharge itself through the VDU operator's body if that person is in close contact with metal objects – like the example of walking across a synthetically carpeted hotel corridor, then touching a metal lift switch. The fingers and indeed sometimes the whole arm can get an electric shock.

In the VDU work terminal the discharge of personal static is often against the chassis of the VDU. Static discharged in this way can interfere with the display or other aspects of the system's operation causing it to 'crash'.

Safety guidelines

Most countries *recommend* that exposure of people to static magnetic fields should not exceed 0.2 tesla for the whole body and 2.0 tesla for the arms and hands if the period is less than fifteen minutes. For prolonged exposure the limits are 0.02 tesla for the whole body and 0.2 tesla for the arms and hands.[27, 28]

In a report produced by the British National Radiological Protection Board, Dr Alaister McKinlay admits that static fields surrounding VDUs not only approach but sometimes exceed the recommended exposure limits.[30]

There is no statutory legislation or meaningful official guideline to warn VDU operators, parents and teachers about the potential dangers to which they might be subjected for up to eight hours daily – and how to avoid unnecessary long and short-term suffering.

Regulatory agencies and manufacturers of hi-tech equipment have considered it unnecessary to investigate the effect on human operators of the static electromagnetic field and the negative ion depletion in the VDU terminal.

It would appear that regulatory agencies and manufacturers who ought to have known better – and felt some responsibility for the unsuspecting 82 million or more people worldwide who are using the equipment – took the attitude that because excess static build-ups in our environment have become commonplace they are therefore now acceptable. It appears to have been decided that the public at large must be prepared to accept the unexpected odd short sharp shock, hoping that the unpleasant and sometimes painful effects of static would pose no seriously harmful long-term consequences – at least none that could be proven. A few years ago I aired my fears on this subject to a spokesman of the National Radiological Protection Board in Leeds. During our conversation he emphatically ensured me:

'There is no dangerous radiation coming from a VDU.'

I asked about static in particular:

'There's no such thing as a static build-up,' he replied. 'If you use an antistatic spray you will get rid of it. There is no evidence that it is harmful.'

That's rubbish and misleading. There *is* a great deal of evidence already, but certainly more tests need to be carried out, most urgently.

Prior to the introduction of computers into our lifestyle there has never been another group of people who spent such prolonged periods being exposed to static of the magnitude which exists in the VDU terminal, or in such close proximity to a high static field – and often for such prolonged periods. Particularly vulnerable are the hands and fingers performing repetitive tasks while surrounded by the strongest source, probably discharging the body's excess static via arms, hands and the fingertips that are in constant and repetitive contact with the keyboard.

Perhaps eventually scientific research will be conducted on static and ion depletion in the VDU environment. When that happens scientists will be able to explain why experienced competent typists, who never suffered RSI injuries whilst using a typewriter keyboard, are suddenly suffering so many new problems whilst sitting in exactly the same positions and doing exactly the same repetitive movements with their fingers on a keyboard with the same QWERTY layout.

To gain some insight into probable detrimental effects we must examine some of the limited amount of research which has been conducted into the problems of static and ion imbalance in non-VDU environments. I am particularly leaving some parts of these edited reports in scientific jargon because it is important to look for the areas where a level of measurements has been reached where there has been no ill effect. It is often at this level that a safety standard is declared – but then at a later date, perhaps, further research conducted well below that safety level will unexpectedly demonstrate that harmful effects are again found to occur, repeating the experience with X-rays and now ELF and VLF.

Research findings

1 The *Hebrew Scientist* reported tests conducted by Dr Sulman into the effects of the depletion of negative ions and the excess of positive ions on pregnant women. When positive ions were increased it was found that the women produced more serotin; once this serotin was in their system the women miscarried. Women who had a record of natural miscarriages were then injected with a serotin blocking agent and almost all then conceived and gave birth to healthy babies. This drug was made illegal in Israel in the mid-sixties.[39]

2 Increased sexual activity has been shown to occur in humans living in an atmosphere which has been artificially charged with negative ions. Testicles and ovaries exposed to high concentrations of negative ions for four days show a stimulation of the maturation process of a large number of cells. On the other hand, those exposed to an atmosphere depleted of negative ions (as in the VDU environment) experienced a suppression of their virility and fertility.[40]

3 Dr Leslie Hawkins, head of the Occupational Health Unit at Surrey University, explains that positive ions in the air get repelled away from the screen on to the operator. When there is a high static field the ion balance in the surrounding air is changed considerably and that can cause many people to feel unwell. They report symptoms of headaches and lethargy in an environment with a build-up of positive ion charges. People are more alert in an environment of negative ions.

4 Dr Charles Wallach of the Faculty of Medicine at the University of California reports that negative ion depletion can affect the sodium/potassium ion exchange in the body which regulates muscular function and this controls fatigue. Negative ion depletion can also affect the calcium ion binding brain tissue, which affects nerve impulses. It inhibits thyroxine conversion (which is a major hormonal process of the thyroid gland) and increases the serum levels of the nerve hormone serotonin which affects the transmission of nerve impulses and has been shown to be responsible for pregnant women losing their babies.[39]

5 Research on animals also indicates that ion depletion has a long-term effect on the mortality of laboratory animals and lowers their resistance to disease.[10, 11]

6 Static combined with negative ion depletion can be the major factor in the now commonly complained of manually crippling tingling sensations in fingers, hands and arms which results from damage to nerve endings. This phenomenon has been well documented in Australia where (after numerous exploratory biopsies) its manifestation is referred to as

'scalloped nerve endings'. Operators often wrongly attribute these problems to RSI (Repetitive Strain Injuries) whereas in fact they are wholly or mostly due to what I have called OSI (Overexposure to Static Injuries).

The problems are compounded by the hindrance or destruction of the natural repair mechanism in the muscles and nerves of the fingers, hands, wrists and arms in particular. There is an urgent need for new research to be conducted to examine the combined effects of static and the depletion of negative ions on the various musculoskeletal and repetitive strain injuries.

7 Tingling sensations in the feet and swelling ankles can be the result of static accumulation at ground level, particularly in those work terminals where static cannot be discharged because of unsuitable floor coverings.

8 There are a number of controlled tests where ionisers have been installed in different offices where VDUs were in use. Because these ionisers emit no noise or visible signs when they are working the VDU operators were not aware if or when they were switched on – putting negative ions in the air. In one such test of eleven weeks' duration (when the ionisers were intermittently working) operators reported feelings of being more calm and alert, enjoying sounder sleep, having more energy, a better appetite, fewer bodily aches and pains, fewer respiratory complaints and having a feeling of wellbeing. There were fewer complaints of nausea and dizziness, while headaches were reduced by 20.6%. There was a 28% improvement in 80% of tasks performed involving accuracy and hand/eye co-ordination.[71]

9 In one Israeli experiment babies cried less when left in a room with high levels of negative ions.[72]

10 Several scientific reports claim that the weak forces exerted on molecules by applied static magnetic fields could alter their kinetic energies or induce conformational changes in enzyme structure, thereby altering biochemical reaction rates.[18-26, 29, 38]

11 There are reports of inhibited growth of cultured cells after exposure to static magnetic fields.[18] Changes in cell metabolism have been observed during exposure *in vitro*. A 20% to 30% depression of oxygen consumption was obtained in embryo mouse kidney and liver tissue during intermittent exposure up to 0.7 tesla.[20] The threshold for these responses was about 0.008 tesla. Surprisingly this depression could not be produced during continuous exposure to 0.6 tesla[21] making the response difficult to interpret. In other words the result of these scientific observations was unexpected, and similar to the ones we looked at earlier in relation to ELF and VLF.

12 Haematological changes have been described in female mice exposed to a static magnetic field of 0.42 tesla for 59 days. Total white blood cell counts in the exposed animals were significantly different from those in the unexposed control group.[22]

13 Various pathological changes have been reported in the Russian literature. For example, morphological changes were seen in guinea pigs

exposed for up to 21 days to static magnetic fields of 0.002 tesla and 0.7
tesla.[23] The severity of the lesions was less at 0.002 tesla but even at this
low field strength transient changes were seen in reproductive organs
(testes), liver, kidneys, adrenals and the lens epithelium.

14 Behavioural and physiological responses have been observed during
acute exposure to more intense fields. Transient changes in behaviour
are described in three squirrel monkeys conditioned to respond to a
visual vigilance task and subsequently exposed to static field of 4.6 to 9.3
tesla. Response rate was greatly suppressed by fields of 7 tesla. Eight
squirrel monkeys trained on several operant tasks showed similar
suppressive effects up to 9.7 tesla. All of these effects were found to be
reproducible.[24]

15 Temporary changes have been detected in electrocardiograms recorded
from squirrel monkeys exposed to between 2 and 7 tesla. An increase in
sinus arrhythmia and a temporary decrease in heart rate was observed
during a three-hour exposure.[25]

16 Several groups of people working in an electrostatic magnetic field have
complained of tooth pains and of a bitter taste in the mouth. These
problems were assumed to be the result of moving the head through a
static magnetic field gradient which induced a current in tooth fillings.[28]

17 Two Russian surveys which monitored 1,329 employees in the machine
building industry exposed at levels between 0.0005 tesla and 0.005 tesla
but reaching a maximum of 0.1 tesla (far below the currently
recommended safety levels) found that they had symptoms which
included headaches, chest pains, rapid development of fatigue, blurred
vision, dizziness, loss of appetite, insomnia, itching, sweating and
burning sensations in the wrists.[27, 29]

These tests were not conducted in a VDU environment and the
employees could additionally have been exposed to other general
pollutants in the atmosphere; it has been suggested that these might
possibly have included airborne metallic dust, various emissions and
degreasing agents which they worked with, or even too high a
temperature in the workplace.

18 Static fields have been shown to affect certain chemical reactions *in vitro*.
Flow potentials will be generated across blood vessels by the flow of
blood perpendicular to the field, but their biological significance at fields
of a few tesla is still not clear.[31]

19 Russian scientists, experimenting on animals and plants, monitored tests
to observe the effects of various levels of negative ions in the air. The
results showed that when there were no negative ions in the atmosphere,
within days the growth in plants was severely stunted and all the animals
died.[185]

20 The static fields attract dust particles and airborne chemical pollutants
which are then deposited on the VDU operator's skin. The pores of the
skin are open and the charged dust penetrates the skin causing blocked
pores, allergies, dermatitis, dryness of skin, skin rashes, eczema and
premature ageing of the skin. The eyes can be affected resulting in
conjunctivitis, dryness and itching.[12, 13]

Faces, necks and hands are prone to the worst suffering because they are exposed the most. In summer, when less and lighter clothing is worn, the symptoms often extend to exposed necks, shoulders and arms. These symptoms usually disappear quite quickly when the operators are away from the VDUs for a few days, only to re-appear with the return to the VDU environment.[2]

21 Assorted skin rashes, premature ageing of the skin, itching eyes and conjunctivitis are common in VDU environments where the electrostatic charge emanating from the VDU is allowed to accumulate which it does if the humidity in the air is not controlled. Not less than 40% relative humidity should therefore be maintained in the air surrounding VDUs.[2, 71]

22 If there is less than 40% or preferably 50% of humidity in the air surrounding the VDU, an electrostatic charge emanating from the screen will accumulate, and this could cause assorted rashes and ageing of the skin in many people,[2] particularly those who have a sensitive skin or those who se skin has a tendency to dryness. Higher humidity helps to eliminate – or at least considerably reduce – the electrostatic charge.[1] Therefore the ideal level of humidity in the surrounding air would be 50%. As that level is reduced the risk of adverse health effects increases – most dramatically if it is allowed to drop to 30% or below.[1, 2, 71]

Time limits and contributory factors

The severity of the problems is linked directly to the amount of time spent in the electrostatically charged environment. These problems can be made considerably worse if combined with other factors – such as a lack of humidity, incorrect ion balance, dust in the air, or other pollutants and additional static increases caused by other office machinery and bad ergonomic design.

Sadly it is often pure vanity which persuades many managements to take steps to spend the money required to protect the well-being of their staff – when they realise that the atmosphere of electronic smog in their own working environment can cause ageing and detrimental effects to their own sexual prowess because of the harmful effects to which their testes and ovaries are exposed.

How to protect yourself

The following will at least considerably reduce – and mostly totally eliminate – unnecessary exposure, and consequently the health risks that result from static fields and negative ion depletion.

1 Use an earthed antistatic screen which fits over the top of, and completely covers, the VDU's own screen. These are designed to protect the person operating the VDU from an excessive build-up of static. They also reduce or eliminate glare and reflections from the screen. They must be cleaned with antistatic chemicals and lint-less cloths. There are two basic kinds of anti-glare screens;

(a) Mesh screens are made from a carbonised cloth which is stretched on to an earthed aluminium frame from a corner of which there is a lead with a clip attached. The principle is that the carbonised cloth collects the static and directs it to the aluminium frame and the thin lead (which must be earthed) directs the static away from operator.

These screens are subject to 'wear', so they can lose their protective properties, sometimes within six months, after which they must be replaced. To find out how much protection you have, the air between the operator and the screen should be regularly checked with an electrostatic locator that measures the exact amount of static that you are exposed to.

(b) Newer, long lasting and more expensive screens are constructed out of glass with an anti-reflective coating, or of tinted and polarised glass with a wired metal surround; they too have a long thin lead attached to the frame which needs to be earthed. Progressive cleaning can damage the anti-reflective coatings on the glass models, while the others are virtually indestructible. However, beware of extravagant claims: some claim variously to eliminate ELF and VLF, or all radiation – that is not only untrue, it is impossible.

There is an enormous difference between the quality and the price of these screens, with a proportionate degree of efficiency. The rule of thumb is; don't buy one until you try it on your screen and have compared the different qualities available. For example, in July 1991 the British prices ranged from £25 for a mesh screen to more than £450 for high quality polarised glass ones.

(c) You have three choices of the way the screen is earthed. At the end of the lead there is a clip; your first choice is to use the clip to grip the head of one of the screws on the back of the casing of the computer – which is itself earthed.

Secondly, you can fix the clip on to the metal of a nearby radiator. The contact must be with metal so if the radiator is painted you would have to scrape the paint away from where the lead is attached.

The disadvantage of these two ways is that the clip can be unknowingly detached or fall off; operators don't realise this has happened, but they have lost all protection. Another point is that it has progressively become good practice to have the computer casing under the desk to create more work space, at the same time lowering the screen to a more acceptable visible level – in which case many leads would not reach the computer casing.

The third, most efficient and reliable choice is to take the clip off the end of the lead and attach the end of the wire firmly to the earth terminal of a three-prong plug which is then connected to the electricity supply in the same way as the plugs on other electrical appliances.

2 Earthed antistatic mats should also be placed beneath the VDU, keyboard and computer on the work-top. There should be a separate one under the printer (which should not be close to the operator). These

mats are available in a variety of sizes ranging from small ones to fit under printers and keyboards alone to quite large ones that will cover most of the work-top. The latter allow plenty of space for the computer, keyboard and sundry equipment, with space to spare so that you can periodically discharge personal static by resting your elbows, forearms and hands on the mat in front of you and alongside the VDU. If you place your hands on the antistatic mat before using the equipment this will take away much of your personal static before the VDU is switched on. Repeat this procedure at intervals whilst using the equipment.

These antistatic mats must also have a lead with a clip which must be earthed as previously described.

3 An added measure of safety is afforded to both operator and equipment by the use of natural fibre carpeting, or a carpet with metal thread woven into it and earthed.

Care must be taken that the carpet is not then placed on top of a synthetically based underfelt, or glued to the floor, because that will stop the static being earthed.

4 If the floor is covered with a carpet constructed wholly or partly from synthetic materials, ensure that it is frequently professionally treated to eliminate static. This should ideally be done every six weeks.

5 Alternatively you can install a separate earthed copper foil grid underneath the operator's chair and the work-top to discharge static build-up.[8]

A wide range of new antistatic mats have recently been introduced to the market – but false claims are attached to some of them; several I have seen carry an 'antistatic' label but they have absolutely no antistatic properties built into them. An antistatic mat must have carbon or some other conducting metallic material woven into it. Efficient ones designed to give protection where the floor is non-conductive have a lead on one edge which is fitted into an electrical plug (as detailed in 1(c) above). A good earthed antistatic floor mat should have a life span of decades, only eventually being visibly worn away by heavy use over a prolonged period.

6 Workers should not wear 'trainer' shoes, because they too can increase static.

7 Check on the humidity of the air in the surrounding area to ensure that the optimum moisture level is maintained. Ideally the level of humidity should be between 40% and 50%; it must never drop below 30%.

8 Choose and wear underwear, outer clothing and shoes made entirely from natural fibres. Because this is necessary for a healthy working environment for the VDU operator perhaps managements could be persuaded to make a contribution towards this. Or do you have a sympathetic member of parliament who can lobby for tax concessions for VDU operators' clothing?

9 Do not perform other tasks with the VDU screen switched on. Switch the VDU off when not actually in use – otherwise it will continue to add unwanted static to the environment around the work terminal. Injuries

and detrimental health effects are suffered in proportion to the time spent in the environment where the VDU screen is continually emitting static into the atmosphere.

10 Take frequent rest breaks of at least ten minutes away from the screen every hour or twenty minutes away from the screen every two hours. Operators should not spend more than four hours in any one day in the vicinity of a live VDU.

11 The static field can be reduced if a shielding box is put round the VDU's case. A shielding box can be constructed simply and cheaply by making a cardboard or plywood box to fit around the top, bottom and two sides of the VDU. The inside of the box is lined with copper foil, with the exception of the areas for ventilation and those are covered with copper mesh screening. A lead is soldered to the casing so that it can then be earthed (as detailed in 2(c)).[14]

Dr Karel Marha, using a field strength meter with plus or minus 0.3% accuracy, found after this case was in position that the static field around it was reduced to zero; all of the static emanating from the flyback transformer was eliminated.[14] Of course the worst emissions – from the screen – were not affected.

12 It is advisable to have professional regular maintenance checks made to monitor the static fields. Static is measured with an 'electrostatic locator'. This device also indicates whether the static is negative or positive. Keep a record of these readings and the dates they are taken.

13 The installation of a filtered negative ioniser in the VDU work terminal is a cheap addition that can bring about major improvements to health and efficiency.

14 Well-watered potted plants can help replace humidity in the air.

15 Vases of fresh flowers also help with replenishing moisture in the air. Additionally, their lifespan will give a graphic illustration of whether or not the VDU working environment is healthy.

I have frequently put fresh cut flowers in various rooms of my home and office, including a display near my VDU. Those near the VDU would die in a few hours whilst the rest look fresh and attractive for a week or more! This was my first sure sign that something was definitely wrong in my own VDU terminal.

16 High temperatures reduce the effectiveness of negative ionisers and worsen the adverse static effects, particularly those of drying and ageing effects on skin. Keeping the temperature down by opening windows is healthier than relying on mechanical air cooling and conditioning units, which are discussed further in Chapter 26.

End note

Worried about the efficiency of my own antistatic screen, I have just asked a service engineer to bring a static meter to check the level. He told me: 'We haven't got any meters, but my fingers are good at detecting static, if it's a problem.'!!!

CHAPTER EIGHTEEN
Synergistic effects

During 1991 the new regulations and laws published in all EC countries will, in keeping with the EC Directive, hold employers responsible for keeping themselves informed of the latest advances in scientific findings about the VDU terminal. Thus enlightened, from the end of 1992 employers will be obliged to perform an analysis of their VDU terminals and make any changes necessary to enable them to guarantee a better level of protection of workers' safety and health.

We have looked at some of the known effects that each of the VDU's different kinds of emitted radiations can have on the body. No matter how low the strength of each of these types of radiation is in any particular VDU terminal, the operator is exposed to them all at the same time, for prolonged periods. These combined effects – in addition to other environmental hazards that exist in the VDU terminal, which are outlined in Part 4 – can cause far more serious health risks than if we were exposed to each kind of radiation individually. This is known as the 'synergistic effect'.

At this stage in the history of the VDU, no one can say exactly what the combined synergistic effects of the VDU's radiation emissions will be on the average sized, healthy body. If the body is not so healthy and there is already an underlying physical weakness, a health problem, or if a person is taking medicines which affect the chemistry of the body, then under any of these circumstances that person might be more susceptible to damage from synergistic effects.

So too would the bodies of children. There is already a great deal of evidence which shows that the bodies of children are more prone to adverse effects from radiation because, whilst they are growing, their bodies are in a process of constant change and are even more vulnerable than those of adults. At this time there is a lamentable lack of studies into what the synergistic effects will be.

We know that the biological effects of radiation are increased when a person is exposed to them with combined high levels of heat or noise. For example, raising the body temperature intensifies the effects of X-ray exposure; that's why cancer patients undergoing X-ray treatments usually have heat packs applied. Damage to body tissues is also greater when exposures to radio frequencies and X-rays occur at the same time. And, if a person is exposed to microwaves that also intensifies the effects of X-ray exposure.[186]

If one part of the body is affected that could alter several other body functions at the same time. We are familiar with the fact that one disease can make your body more susceptible to another infection or weakness. For example, liver disease affects virtually every organ in the body.[88] A combination of radiations have been seen to affect the body's reaction to chemical substances, both from the environment and those swallowed, including a wide range of prescribed medicines.[187]

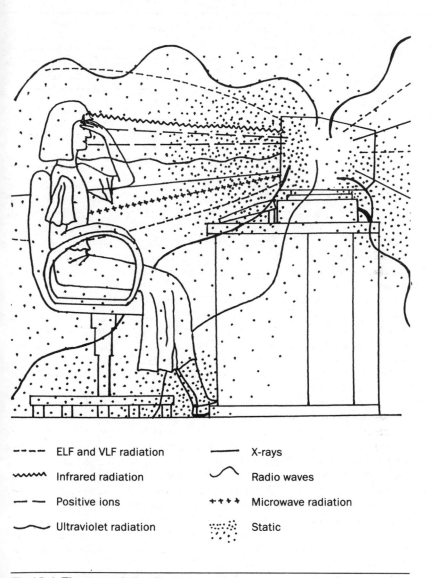

---- ELF and VLF radiation	—— X-rays
ᗰᗰᗰ Infrared radiation	⌒ Radio waves
— — Positive ions	++++ Microwave radiation
⌒⌒ Ultraviolet radiation	∴∷∴ Static

Fig 18.1 The synergistic effects

Whilst I was writing this chapter the insurance policy on my own VDU came up for renewal. I was interested even if a little alarmed to find, in the small print, that they exclude insurance cover for any problems relating to radiation! This clause I am assured is normal.

PART FOUR

Ergonomics: The study of workers and the working environment

CHAPTER NINETEEN
There is going to be a revolution

There is going to be a revolution! New legislation which comes in force at the end of 1992 will make manufacturers and employers accountable for providing safer equipment and environmental facilities for VDU operators. They will also be accountable for the health problems suffered by VDU users. Employers will be obliged to keep themselves informed of the latest advances in technology – and scientific findings – and make any changes necessary so as to be able to *guarantee* a better level of protection of workers' safety and health.[1]

It is easy to understand the unpleasant and unhealthy working conditions in the factories of yesteryear. Threatening voluminous clouds of black smoke belched out of factory chimneys polluting surrounding towns and countryside. Harsh concrete floors and brick walls stained with oil, grease and dirt were almost impossible to clean. Working conditions within austere dark walls were noisy, cold, drafty and dirty. Employees performed laborious work in cramped conditions for over-long working hours. You could *see, hear, smell, touch and feel* the old problems.

There are more numerous and serious health problems in contemporary clean, energy-efficient, but chemically and electrically polluted hi-tech city offices and schools than there were in the old dark satanic mills and sweat shops.

Surrounding today's unsuspecting smartly dressed professionals and office staff are new health risks that they don't feel. The sources are mostly invisible, quiet and odourless. Nobody is more exposed and at risk than VDU users.

If we work a physically strenuous regular ten-hour day we accept that we might feel tired, listless and irritable and develop muscular aches and pains. Comparatively few hours spent in a sedentary position in light, bright, clean buildings – or sitting at the home computer – can have worse health effects if the working practices, ambient air, furnishings and accessories have not been acquired and designed specifically for VDU work.

Collectively, futuristic hi-tech pioneers have invented unhealthy manufactured air in energy-conserving buildings designed with big, sealed, light-reflecting windows.[2]

Inside are unsuitable decorations, inappropriate old electrical systems and furnishings that are relics of a bygone era. Fluorescent lights flickering at 50 cycles per second can interfere with human brain-wave patterns and sometimes drip poisonous PCBs. The bare old ordinary tungsten house bulb is far superior.

Additionally there might be inappropriate futuristic shapes of furniture dreamed up by designers who have neither practical nor well researched knowledge about the effects of the physical interactions of sedentary humans working with or near hi-tech equipment.[3,4]

Beware the new buzz word 'ergonomic design'. It is being wrongly and misleadingly used by hundreds of manufacturers and salespeople to describe chairs, desks and light fittings that have absolutely no ergonomic benefits whatsoever. The interesting thing about the word 'ergonomics' is that it is neutral. It's the study of the relationship between the worker and his/her working environment. So when a manufacturer says a chair is 'ergonomic', they're not really saying much; the question is whether it is ergonomically *good* or *bad*! By the time you have finished reading this book you will know whether these claims are true or false.

Then, there is the electronic equipment itself which frequently has manufacturing defects and/or has been badly installed.[5] Added to which, little, if any, consideration has been given to the pre-planning of entirely new working practices and routines which themselves necessitate revolutionary new 'in-house' facilities.

Millions of VDU operators from three continents and over fifty different countries have a common list of health complaints that international epidemiologists have attributed to ergonomic problems (inappropriate working methods and badly designed working environments).[6] These complaints include: abdominal cramps, alveolitis, asthma, bladder problems, blurred vision, bowel problems, bronchitis, chronic catarrh, chronic fatigue, depression, deterioration in muscles, tendons and joints, digestive complaints, disturbances of colour vision, disturbed sleep patterns, dizziness, dry and itching eyes, eye strain, fatigue in the retina which affects peripheral vision, an assortment of gastric troubles, headaches, heart disease, haemorrhoids, humidifier fever, indigestion, irregular disrupted menstrual patterns, irritability, legionnaires disease, lethargy, loss of appetite, loss of control of eye movements which lead to disorientation, loss of sexual drive, migraines, miscarriages, muscular and circulatory problems in legs, muscular problems in arms, wrists, fingers, back, head, neck, and shoulders, nausea, nervous disorders, pontiac fever, postural problems, repetitive strain injuries, reproductive problems, rheumatic problems, stress, sinusitis, tension, tiredness and varicose veins.

Under the Health and Safety at Work Act 1974 employers in the UK have a duty to provide safe equipment, safe methods of work, information and instruction, safe workplaces (in terms of the amount of space, layout, electrical installations, access and egress), and a safe working environment (lighting, heating, noise and ventilation). Additionally the Offices Shops and Railway Premises Act sets out minimum standards on space, temperature, ventilation, lighting and seating for sedentary work. Many of today's schools, universities and offices do not meet the old minimum standards set out in these two acts. Neither of these two pieces of legislation specifically covers the circumstances of VDU operators.

According to the Orbit study about 80% of London's leased offices are inadequately designed and equipped to support hi-tech office automation.[7]

In America it is estimated that 150 million working days are lost yearly through illness related to the sick building syndrome.

A leading scientist from the World Health Organisation says, 'There is probably more damage to human health by indoor pollution than outdoor pollution.'[18]

Canada, Japan, Australia, and several European countries, especially those with socialised medicine – and thus a real fiscal interest in the long-term health hazards of new technology – have already adopted new standards for regulating VDUs, their use, and the use of terminal support furniture. America, lacking that financial incentive, has failed so far to follow the lead of Germany, Sweden, France and others. Britain, instead of following the responsible lead of her European neighbours, seems to have adopted the policy that if the Americans can get away with it so can we, possibly paving the way for a rash of product liability lawsuits in the next decade, according to a spokesperson for NIOSH, the Atlanta-based National Institute for Occupational Safety and Health.[8]

- Scandinavian countries have already issued special directives, guidelines and laws governing the use of VDUs. Sweden even provides approved technical specifications for the equipment used and the work station design. These countries have implemented regulations governing work station facilities and furniture, physical checks for operators and restricted working time. There is also an order governing the ergonomics of movement and posture in the workplace relating to VDU work.[9]
- Similar standards adopted in Austria have additionally designated VDU work carried out at night as falling within the special protective regulations for night workers.[10]
- France has designated VDU work as falling within those occupations requiring special regular surveillance by occupational medical specialists.[11]
- Australia states that radiation hazards do exist. They set out ergonomic design considerations for equipment and the work station. Preventative measures include regular rest breaks.[12]
- Japan's official guidelines include regular physical examination, training, rest breaks, maximum working hours and pre-placement consideration.[13]

■ Canadian regulations stipulate relocation away from VDUs for pregnant operators, ergonomic design, frequent rest breaks, five-hour maximum daily work time and medical checks,[14] along with low levels of non-ionising radiation emissions from VDUs,[15] stress control measures and eye tests.[16]

The problems surrounding your VDU

These problems fall into five main categories that are easy to understand and deal with. These are additional to the radiation problems.

1 Personal organisation and new working practices designed to eliminate or minimise health hazards specific to using the VDU.
2 Lack of the requisite sundry equipment and facilities necessary for the safe operation of the VDU.
3 Electropollution (combined radiation risks of all the equipment) present in the terminal in addition to those caused by the VDU itself.
4 Space allocation and office planning where the VDU is installed. It is possible that although the equipment is good problems will occur because it is badly sited, decorations, furnishings or the power supply are unsuitable, or the space is too cramped.
5 The sick building syndrome.

How to organise your working practices and protect yourself

1 The checklists in this book give details of all the various safety measures to be taken in the different aspects of the work terminal. If you are not self-employed you need to know that your employer fulfills all the responsibilities outlined. Under the new EC rules ignorance is no excuse. Employers now have a responsibility to keep themselves up-to-date with new technical and scientific information as that becomes available. Employers will be paying a salary for your labour – not for risking your health either long or short term.
2 Some of the health problems originating in the VDU terminal will be apparent at the time they are caused. Several others will take varying lengths of time to develop before symptoms become obvious.

   Some makes and models of VDUs have been shown to be more harmful than others – and that will undoubtedly continue to be true of future models.

   It would be wise to keep a record of the make, model number, and serial numbers (printed on the casing) of the VDUs, keyboards and other electronic equipment that you either use, or that are located close to you.
3 From the outset a contract between employer and employee (or student) is vital. It must:
   (a) ensure that you are not expected to work either with or near a switched on VDU for more than two consecutive hours, or for an

absolute maximum of four hours in any one day, or twenty hours in any week; and that adequate rest breaks away from the screen are provided during that time.

(b) specify what type of regular eye and medical checks are available, with a doctor of the employee's choice, at the employer's expense.

(c) give young women who are contemplating becoming or have become pregnant the right to be moved away from the VDU to work on other jobs at a parallel level. For example, new guidelines outlaw the practice of banishing pregnant women VDU operators to washing dishes or performing other tasks unrelated to existing occupational ability, experience and salary structure.

(d) if and when new items are introduced to the VDU workplace, give the employee the right to professional training before operating the equipment or software. Even some of the more complex chairs and lights need to be carefully explained if somebody is to gain the maximum benefit from them.

(e) inform the VDU operator that efficient 'hot-line' facilities are available on all the software packages.

(f) provide the operator with details of servicing and maintenance arrangements for VDUs and other hi-tech equipment that he or she will be required to use or that will be located in the nearby working environment. In relation to VDUs the service contract must include at least twice-yearly measurements of each of the different types of electromagnetic radiation emitted and the levels of static surrounding the equipment, as well as the right to call out a maintenance engineer when the VDU develops a problem, breaks down completely, or for cleaning purposes.

Operators should always keep their own copies of these readings (along with the dates and serial numbers of equipment used).

(g) give VDU operators a right to know about all electrical or hi-tech items and equipment introduced into the environment which they themselves might not use but that may overload the body's exposure to radiation.

Because of the nature of some of the radiation emitted by the VDU it is possible for someone from outside the organisation to tune into the radio waves from the VDU you are working on – and steal what might be highly confidential information.

For security reasons some companies have introduced descramblers which disrupt the electromagnetic radiation coming off your VDU, making it impossible for an outsider to pick up the information. Descramblers often emit more harmful radiation than the VDU itself. So, if a descrambler is installed close to you, your radiation exposure level is considerably increased.

Every additional piece of electrical equipment is capable of having some effect on your body. If one single 100 watt bulb is switched on in the room, although you are completely unaware of any physical effect, your brain's electroencephalogram rhythms immediately change.[17]

4 Some form of daily exercise is vital to counteract the physically debilitating effect of sedentary work – even if you only walk briskly for twenty minutes each day. I would suggest yoga and swimming to keep the spine supple but it really must be a personal choice depending on your preferences and physical condition.

   Larger, caring firms are now providing health studios offering a range of physical activities and equipment. For less energetic members of staff medically approved passive-exercise beds are provided: you just lie there whilst the mechanisms stimulate circulation and muscles as they stretch, strengthen and straighten the spine.

5 Wearing leather shoes and clothes made out of natural fibres will help reduce adverse radiation effects in the terminal.

6 Are you worth £2.5 million? Know your value! It is extremely expensive to provide a safe working environment for everyone who uses a VDU. Those who cannot or will not spend time in understanding the problems and money to make the environment safe, should quite simply never install a VDU in the first place. That applies equally to the self-employed, parents, and schools, as it does to both small and large companies employing staff.

   Although justifiable on humanitarian grounds alone, there are very real financial considerations. For example, if a 20-year-old enters a company at a salary of £10,000 per annum, works there for thirty years, receives an 8% annual increase, retires at half salary and lives to the age of 75 – that person represents a £2.5 million investment to the company.[7] For a person reaching top management the figure can be ten times that figure.

   If a company, a parent, a teacher, or a self-employed person had a machine worth that kind of money they'd build a fence around it, polish it, show it off and have someone specially trained to supply its needs. People need to be treated with the same level of respect for the investment they represent.

   In the following pages we get down to the nitty-gritty of the planning and subsidiary items needed to keep us healthy when we use the VDU.

CHAPTER TWENTY
Essential subsidiary equipment

Several extra bits and pieces of equipment ought to be supplied with the VDU but usually are not – even though they are absolutely vital in making the VDU function in an efficient and compatible way with humans.

Antistatic desk mat

In the days of the typewriter, each and every one of them came complete with a thick rubber-topped felt mat that absorbed vibrations and allowed the machine to be easily moved about on the work surface. VDUs are usually supplied without this facility. Nonetheless a different type of mat should be placed beneath every VDU.

The VDU mat should be of the antistatic type with a lead which is itself connected to the earth terminal of a three-pin plug, then plugged into the mains electricity supply so that it is properly earthed. This helps to protect the operator from the ever-present static field surrounding the VDU.

Antistatic floor mat

The principle is the same as the desk mat. It must be similarly earthed to make it effective. The size should be not less than 1200 mm wide by treble the depth of the work-top so that the chair can easily be moved around without the operator losing protection.

I was recently horrified to see an alternative solution, whereby the operator wore a sort of ankle bracelet which was then earthed to the electric supply. Hopefully no-one who reads this book will allow themselves to be so dangerously chained to the office desk!

Dust cover

It is surprising but true that dust does not settle on the VDU screen whilst it is switched on. When the VDU is switched off dust is attracted to the screen. You have probably noticed that your domestic TV screen holds far more dust than the surrounding furnishings in your room do. As soon as the VDU is switched on an electrical charge blasts all the dust off the screen on to the operator's face. Not just dust, but dust combined with static and positive ions. The result; blocked pores, spots, red blotches and dry irritated skin and dry eyes, in sensitive people. So the VDU screen should be covered at all times when it is not being used.

VDU manufacturers' cost-cutting practices invariably omit the inclusion of this important item when they sell the VDU.

Tilt and swivel stand

The vertical and horizontal angles of a VDU screen must be adjustable. You must be able to swivel it from side to side and tilt it up or down to whatever angle is best suited to your working conditions and personal preferences.

Some VDUs have this facility built-in, others do not. In the latter case a separate tilt and swivel stand must be bought and the VDU placed upon it.

Faraday cage

VDU casing should be metal with a matt decorative finish. If you are unfortunate enough to be presented with a plastic case then a protective metal surround (a Faraday cage) must be ordered from your service engineer to protect you from as much of the radiation as possible.

You can protect yourself in this way from the electric field but you can not escape the magnetic field. The only protection you have from the magnetic field is to move away completely from the offending field, or switch the equipment off.[1]

Take care that ventilation is not blocked if a protective casing has to be supplied separately. Ventilation should be directed upwards, or situated on the back of the casing, so that it does not direct noxious emissions directly onto the VDU operator.

Hard disk stand and extension cables

In the case of personal computers the VDU frequently stands on top of the computer casing that houses the floppy disk drive and hard disk. It is preferable that this piece of the equipment is located in a separate mobile computer stand which is placed within arm's reach, on the floor, alongside the work-top. Otherwise, besides taking up valuable work-top space, it raises the level of the screen to a height that often necessitates the head being tilted slightly backwards putting pressure on nerves and muscles in the neck. (The most beneficial physical position allows the head to remain in the normal upright position whilst the eyes should look straight ahead or slightly down to the screen. You should never use a screen if you have to look up to it.)

These stands come with or without castors. Mobility is essential so that the computer can be easily and safely moved for cleaning and convenient re-positioning. When ordering a hard disk stand you will also need to buy extension cables long enough to reach it.

Document holder

A heavy-weighted solid based document holder that allows papers and files to be viewed at the same eye level as the screen is required to avoid a bent body posture over the work-top – which often results in muscular problems in the neck and back. The document holder must be large enough to hold the shape, size and thickness of papers or books referred to whilst operating the VDU. It must also be adjustable in height and tilt so that it can be positioned to suit the individual operator's working practices and eyesight. It should preferably be at the same height, angle and distance from the operator as the VDU screen.

Footstool

If the height of the work-top necessitates the seat of the chair being raised to a level where the entire soles of the feet do not comfortably rest on the floor, then a footstool is necessary so that the correct posture can be achieved without strain or discomfort. There is no similarity between a VDU footstool and the little Victorian footstool on which, long ago, madam displayed her ankle by the fireside.

New regulations stipulate that the VDU footstool must have a minimum of length of 1200 mm to extend the whole length of the free leg-space beneath the work-top. The top of the footstool must be adjustable in height up to 50 mm, and have a 20 degree tilt facility[1-4] to facilitate individual needs.

Ioniser

A small personal ioniser on the desk can reap huge benefits to most people in promoting feelings of alertness, efficiency and well-being. The static surrounding the VDU depletes the air of negative ions and leaves us with more harmful positive ions. A small desk-top personal ioniser will redress this problem.

Plants

Some plants are said to absorb radiation and/or chemical pollutants from the atmosphere whilst other plants will be adversely affected by the radiation, with changes in their colouring, structure and health alerting us to the invisible radiation problems in the VDU terminal. According to research by NASA (the US National Aeronautics and Space Administration) the green spider plant has proved most effective in getting rid of carbon monoxide, the philodendron at absorbing formaldehyde from carpeting and building materials which can cause flu-like symptoms, species of daisy and chrysanthemums clean up cigarette and paint fumes and counteract benzine from office solvents and some types of felt-tip pen, along with other toxic vapours – because tiny openings in the plants' leaves remove harmful substances directly from the air. They work most efficiently if fans are placed nearby.

I have neither seen research data nor heard claims about assessing health hazards in the VDU terminal from fresh-cut flowers but, as I mentioned earlier, I have frequently found that roses placed near my own VDU die within hours whilst those cut at the same time live for days and sometimes weeks in adjoining computer-less rooms. 'Something' in the VDU terminal exterminates them.

Eye specialists recommend a plant or flowers to provide a focal point to look at so that we are conscious of the necessity to periodically exercise or rest the eyes – away from the screen.

Screen filters

Because of the nature of the VDU it is not unreasonable to expect that they are all supplied with non-reflective and antistatic facilities built into them. They are not. This is therefore another essential 'add-on' which must be bought separately.

The quality of VDU screens varies considerably between manufacturers. Some are more prone to problems of reflection and glare than others. If the VDU screen was designed to polarise the light in one direction and a secondary screen designed to cross polarise was placed beyond that (between the first screen and the worker) there would be no glare. To achieve this it is necessary to buy a separate polarising-glass screen.

By far the best solution is to have a detachable, earthed antistatic, polarising-glass screen, so that glare, reflections and static are dealt with at the same time.[19] Detailed instructions on fitting and earthing these are given in Chapter 17.

Ensure that the antistatic screen is checked for effectiveness every three months, or sooner if you feel that it has lost its efficiency. A survey in Sweden found that eight months after installing these filters 87% of them had ceased to give any protection whatsoever. The manufacturers suggested that the reason might possibly be that incorrect cleaning routines had led to the destruction of the conducting layer.[5] This is particularly relevant to the mesh screen.

The keyboard

I have already dealt with the main principles of the keyboard in Chapter 3.

1 The VDU keyboard must stand alone as a separate unit so that its position and angle on the work-top suits the individual operator. Older models and most lap-top computers that have the keyboard attached to the screen are a common source of RSI, muscular and eye problems.
2 The underside of the keyboard must have adjustable feet so that the tilt can be altered, giving operators the freedom to choose the keyboard angle most suitable to them.
3 Ergonomists say that the most restful position of arms and hands occurs when the angle at the elbow is 90 degrees, so that the forearm and wrists maintain the natural position which they have when the arms are loosely by the side of the body in the natural standing position – wrists neither bent up nor down.
4 The chiropractic view is that, in practice, the comparatively steeply sloping drawing boards of architects and draughtsmen afford the least stressful muscular position. This most nearly approximates to the sharp upward tilt of the old typewriter keyboards – whose operators did not complain of RSI and muscular problems.

Wrist support

A recent addition to the accessories markets is a low padded stand designed to support the wrists of operators who are doing continual data-entry work on a low or flat keyboard. It is placed on the desk top in front of the keyboard. The manufacturers claim that this helps to reduce aching wrists and RSI symptoms. At this time I can find no evidence to support these claims.

Task lighting

Every VDU operator requires a special desk-based light to give added controll-able intensity and directional light on to papers and documents used on the work-top. The design features required of the task light are detailed fully in Chapter 25.

Clean power

The VDU does not work happily off the mains electricity supply, which is referred to in the trade as 'dirty power'. Some geographical areas – and some countries – are worse than others. Just as there is little point in selling an electric kettle without a lead and plug to a person with no electricity, and just as manufacturers of professional photographic colour enlargers always include voltage stabilisers with their equipment, so too should VDU manufacturers ensure that this vital piece of equipment is included in the package. Sadly, it never is.

The operator needs to know from what source clean power is supplied to the VDU. In most smaller offices, and for the home computer user, a desk-based voltage stabiliser or uninterrupted power supply will need to be added to the equipment, to protect both it and the operator. This matter is dealt with fully in the next chapter.

CHAPTER TWENTY-ONE
The mains power supply

The design of the electricity supply will affect the safety of the equipment and the amount of heat generated. It will also determine the amount and the characteristics of radiation that you are exposed to.

We are not supplied with a reliable or constant flow of clean, stable electricity from the national grid. Fluctuating voltages are something we have learned to put up with unquestioningly over the years. The average power loss in the UK in 1984 worked out at almost two hours per customer. That figure includes over 23 million different interruptions lasting over sixty seconds each – and that does not include the purely local or in-house glitches caused by blown fuses, heavy demand and so on.

We have all seen the room lighting suddenly dim, or heard the fridge or some other piece of electrical equipment develop an occasional odd sound or vibration, because of a change in the voltage. Cooks will remember occasions when carefully timed recipes turned out to be disappointingly over or under cooked – not due to faulty timing or lack of care on the part of the cook but because, unknown to us, the voltage of the power supply to our homes was either higher or lower than it ought to have been to enable the cooker to work at its intended performance. Reduced voltages also lower the efficiency of room heaters, hairdryers and so on, and can prevent fluorescent lights from working at all.

A contributing factor is that fluctuations of demand for electricity occur whenever high power consuming equipment is switched on – like industrial plants, central heating boilers, air conditioning systems, lifts, etc. These may be anywhere within the district where our supply comes from, as well as within our individual building.

Most of the electrical equipment of yesteryear was tolerant of these spikes and surges of voltage fluctuations. Today's computers (along with quite a lot of other highly sensitive electronic equipment such as photographic colour enlargers) are not built to tolerate this erratic behaviour from our mains electricity supply.

When one of these highs or lows of voltage supply occurs the computer and its VDU behave erratically and sometimes dangerously. They can considerably increase its radiation emissions. Unpredictably, the computer can lose the information in its memory and the work in progress.

Pulsating vibrations can occur. The work on the screen could appear to lock completely, nothing can be moved, and work certainly cannot continue. Unfamiliar messages can appear on the screen, warning buzzers can sound, or the VDU can simply black out completely. Alternatively the screen may begin jittering or flashing with effects varying from stressful and annoying to catastrophic for the hardware, the work in the computer and particularly and most importantly for the operator.

The hazards we and our sensitive equipment are exposed to include:

Spikes These are dramatic unpredictable jumps in power (such as a strike by lightning). As many as 6,000 volts can zap through your system – enough to permanently damage your computer hardware.

Surges and sags These are slower and less powerful than spikes. They can be caused by switching on or off a nearby electrical appliance which creates an over-voltage (or under-voltage) that can scramble data and distort the programmes on the computer.

Noise This is like the interference you can get on a radio set (often caused by a buzzing fluorescent light). Unless filtered out it can cause screen interference, corrupt data or cause read/write errors.

Fluctuations Circuit-switching at your local power station can create surges and brief interruptions that can fool the VDU into thinking that it is experiencing a power failure. The result? Lost data – any time!

Blackouts A complete loss of power (no matter how brief) can completely destroy the working programmes and information stored on disk.

Whenever one of the above phenomena occurs, the VDU cannot be classed to be in perfect working order. Sometimes the VDU will resume its operation without the attention of a repair or maintenance engineer. But an internal component may have become partially damaged and therefore the VDU can now have become a potential risk with altered radiation levels.

Authoritative and regulatory bodies aim to minimise these problems and pacify workers by stating variously that these electrical variations happen only where there is a particularly high concentration of industry, or in quieter areas which might be served with their electricity supply via sub-station. Let's be realistic; that covers almost every geographical area where the VDU might be used.

Voltage stabilisers and uninterrupted power supplies

In order to protect the operator's health and efficiency, the equipment and the work stored within its system, it is essential that the computer system is supplied with an absolutely guaranteed consistent clean supply of power which is not shared by other items of equipment.

One of the many uninterrupted power stabilising systems must be installed – as they are in government departments and by the more responsible, larger, prosperous companies, many of whom now have their own generating systems.

Most computer equipment supply companies now stock a range of suitable equipment, known as UPSs (uninterrupted power supplies), to carry out this task. They will vary in size, ranging from the smallest which will protect the single installation of one personal computer to large models catering for many more units.

What every VDU operator needs to know is whether or not the equipment they are using is adequately protected by a UPS of the correct size.

This is one of the areas where schools and employers often cut the costs of safety. For, to give adequate protection the requisite UPS can cost as much as the basic hardware of some of the cheaper computers. People looking for the cheapest way to take advantage of computers often neglect to buy this necessary additional piece of equipment, exposing the operator to unnecessary health risks and frustrations.

CHAPTER TWENTY-TWO
The chair, the desk and power at your finger-tips

Before backache was commonplace and it became the accepted thing to spend most of our working lives sitting, desk-bound people used not to have the musculoskeletal problems increasingly suffered today. Many of the 'oldies' like Winston Churchill, Victor Hugo and Ernest Hemingway used to spend much of their time standing at high, sloping work-tops.[7]

The inter-relationship between the chair and desk must not be complementary only to each other, but also to the stature of the person using them and to the type of work being done.

In 1981 the EC committee for standardisation (CEN) sent out for approval new standards for office furniture. The new lower recommended height for tables was 720 mm for all non-adjustable tables. CEN gave no explanation, nor did it publish the names of the persons responsible for this idea. Furniture designers and manufacturers accepted these guidelines unquestioningly.[1-3]

Two years later at the world conference on Ergonomics and Health in Modern Offices held in Turin in 1983, Denmark's chief surgeon A.C. Mandal particularly drew attention to the CEN recommendations. He said:

Man's average height has increased by 10 cm during the last century but for some incomprehensible reason the height of tables has decreased by about 10 cm. The natural consequence of this is that we have to sit more bent over. To sit like this for many hours every day produces a long-term strain on the bones, tendons and muscles of the spine.

Backache has become a serious problem all over the industrialised world and nothing will strain the back for nearly as long a time as the fact that we spend a good deal of our time hunched over tables that are too low, whilst at the same time sitting on inappropriate seating. If you base prevention of backache on the CEN illusions you are doomed to fail.[4]

Within five years his predictions had become reality. Yet today, with continually rising figures for back problems and absenteeism, most office and school furniture designers and manufacturers do not heed the medical opinions and recommendations.

The chair

A chair of the correct dimensions with total adjustability is absolutely vital to the health and well-being of VDU operators, and far more so than to any other sector of workers. Because of the diversity of tasks performed, both VDU and non-VDU work, and because of the limitations of even the best chairs available, perhaps the solution would be for operators to have two quite different chairs.

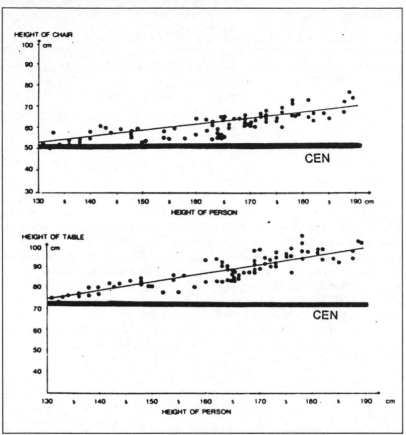

Fig 22.1 Preferred height of chair and table (marked ●). CEN recommendation marked by solid line. (Tables supplied by A. C. Mandal.)

Operators sitting on inappropriate chairs, in a radiation-polluted atmosphere, performing repetitive tasks with static loading on bones, muscles and nerves, *will* suffer from a host of physical and stress-related problems.

The chair must *perfectly* hold, support and move with the body.

Prolonged sitting on inappropriate seating for long periods of time can have adverse effects on the abdominal area, and create disc problems in the spine and neck; colon and bowel problems; stomach cramps; indigestion; and menstrual disorders and miscarriages.

Inappropriate seating positions and space cause problems with diminished blood flow to areas supporting body weight; circulation in legs, knees and feet; and musculoskeletal problems in the back, neck, shoulders, and arms. Unsuitable seating also contributes to stress and to general debility.

The status of the chair

Nothing is more inappropriate, or amusing, than the categories of chairs in manufacturers' brochures. Chairs are quite clearly sold as status symbols. The catalogues clearly demonstrate this point as they categorically differentiate between executive chairs, secretarial/VDU operators' seating and guest chairs.

Corporate seniority and salary structure determine both the size, flexibility and the quality of upholstery. No account is taken of the physical size of the individual who is to sit on a chair, the length of time it is in continual use, or the type of work being done.

I recently visited the ergonomically conscious chairman of a large public company. His tall willowy secretary led me into his spacious and beautifully furnished, thickly carpeted prestigious office. During the few minutes I waited for him to arrive I admired his enormous, highly polished rosewood desk whose tidy spacious surface was broken only by a couple of closed files, a marble futuristic light and an expensive executive toy. My eyes roamed over matching book shelves, cupboards and drawers and a couple of strategically hung pictures – one a hunting scene, the other a yacht in full sail on a rough sea. Below the high ceiling concealed cornice lights ran round the perimeter of the room with four concealed and diffused ceiling lights placed away from, but parallel to, the desk and windows. Bright sunlight was cleverly diffused by vertical slatted blinds covering the large slightly opened windows.

The *pièce de résistance* had to be his very large, sturdy, dark-green leather upholstered, flexibly mobile, ergonomically designed chair. This was the epitome of the perfect office for 'the big man'. Masculine and powerful.

Within minutes I was honoured with his presence when, dressed in a dark grey, immaculately tailored light wool suit he strode purposefully across the room and firmly shook my hand before perching his agile short frame on the edge of his big impressive chair!

No way were his legs long enough to allow him to sit back in this masterpiece of seating, with his bum at the back of the chair so that his spine could be properly supported. Not unless he adopted the lotus or cross-legged position! The depth of the impressive seat wouldn't allow the knees of his little legs to bend so that his feet could touch the floor. Moreover, scatter cushions, to fill empty inches twixt spine and chair-back, are simply not on in these circumstances. Fortunately, shrewd designers and salesmen can partly overcome these problems by introducing a forward tilt to the seat and by placing a discrete footstool (hidden from the prying eyes of staff and guests) behind the floor-length courtesy panelling on the front of the desk – thus elevating the top man to, almost, fit the top seat.

After our meeting ended I passed the tall willowy secretary in her well designed spacious VDU work-terminal. Regrettably, although sitting with her back supported properly and her bum placed at the back of the pink-leather ergonomically designed VDU operator's chair, the depth of the seat was far too small for her long legs. A recipe for circulatory and muscle problems in the legs and feet.

Just as you cannot buy a standard sweater and expect it to perfectly fit every male and female employee doing the same job, the same principle applies to the chair. It is simply not possible for offices to standardise on one particular design and model of chair to suit all VDU operators who, as any fashion designer will tell you, come in a multiplicity of shapes and sizes.

There are three different points of view as to what constitutes the perfect chair. The best thing to do to appreciate the differences is to visit a local office supplier to test all the chairs until you find the right one for you – so that when you buy your own, or approach the boss, you know what you are talking about.

Design criteria relied upon by manufacturers

There is a worldwide unanimity of opinions from furniture manufacturers with respect to 'correct' sitting posture, namely that the spine should be upright, and the feet on the floor. Here are the salient points relied upon.

1 The operator's back should be erect so that it can be supported from the base of the spine to at least shoulder blade level.

2 The lower part of the chair back must be contoured to fit and support the natural curve of the lumbar region. Therefore, the angle between thigh and spine must be 90 degrees.

3 The chair back must also have a back-tilt facility of up to 25 degrees. This is to allow the operator to periodically recline in a relaxing position while the operator's feet and the entire base of the chair must remain on the floor.

   With loss of dignity and the risk of a fall, some people tilt their chair back on two legs and put their feet on the desk, subconsciously trying to compensate for inadequate seating and poor chair design.

4 There must be a locking device within hands' reach of the seated person, located either under the seat or on the chair back, so that the chair back can be readjusted or locked into position at the appropriate angle to support the back in the most comfortable position whilst the VDU operator is performing physically static keyboard tasks.

5 The angle at the knees should also be 90 degrees so that feet are placed flat on the floor.

6 The correct seat height for any operator is again determined by the 90 degree angle at the knees. Therefore the height of the chair must be adjustable.

   Instead of the old system of swivelling the chair seat around to wind the height up or down, today this action is performed at the touch of a button, via a gas cylinder in the base of the chair. This should be regularly checked and serviced. There have been occasions in the past where these gas-lift metal columns have suddenly exploded causing injury and on one occasion death. Modern chairs have an inner casing which protects against this. Be sure yours has one.

7 There must be no pressure on the thighs from the chair seat. A soft shaped *waterfall edge* on the front of the seat prevents this problem. The front edge of the chair must never be hard because that can restrict circulation in the legs – and press on the sciatic nerve if the seat is too long from front to back.

8 The *length* of the chair seat must be long enough to support the body from buttocks to about three inches away from the back of the knees, so that the sciatic nerve cannot be pressed.
9 The *base* of the chair must be solid and firm with *five legs*, each with a castor for mobility.
10 Finally the fabric used for the upholstery should be a natural fibre.

Personal experiences

1 I found that on many, otherwise excellent, chairs loaned to me, the seat could not be lowered sufficiently for my feet to sit squarely on the floor. I am not tall – a mere 163 cm (5' 4") – nonetheless there are a lot of women who work with VDUs who are far shorter than I am. Therefore the claims that these chairs suited 90% of the population were ill-founded.
2 If you are shorter than 173 cm (5' 8") another problem invariably arises relating to desk heights being too high. If this is a problem the situation is to use a height-adjustable 1200 mm long foot stool.
3 Three outstanding ergonomically designed chairs with multidirectional versatility, support and comfort, are the Giroflex 44 (particularly the pyramid model for VDU workers), and the Lingas, both manufactured by Gordon Russell,[19] along with the Sensor by Steelcase Strafor.[20]
4 It can take quite a determined mental and physical effort to correct bad seating postures adopted over the years. Perhaps the chairs should have seat belts fitted to hold us in place initially. On many occasions, I have noticed employees working for chair manufacturers sitting on well-designed chairs who did not sit back on the seats to gain any benefit whatsoever from the inherent design. It took me several days, or even weeks, of concentrated effort to sit in the approved position. Once I had mastered the technique – whilst doing straight keyboard work – I did feel a very definite benefit. But not for desk-based research, when I need to refer to a great many documents on the desk, and when maintaining a straight spine is a physical impossibility. All of these ergonomically designed chairs lacked the flexibility to deal with this common problem.
5 If you find that the 90 degree angles between spine and thigh, or at the knee, uncomfortable, or an impossibility to maintain, you will find an alternative position discussed on page 147.

Medical opinions

Tommy Hansson, head of orthopaedic surgery at Sahlgren Hospital in Sweden, says it has been found that both the intradiscal pressure (pressure in the discs of the spine) and the back muscle activity are reduced when a back rest is used and especially when it is tilted from upright to 110 degrees so that it carries a bigger proportion of the body load. The height of the back rest must extend to the level of the shoulder blades.

Further reduction of both disc pressure and muscular activities is obtained by adding a contoured lumbar support in the back rest and arm rests. Supporting your arms on the desk can offer similar relief to that experienced with arm rests.[5]

Dr Scott Middleton, a chiropractor of radio and television fame, decries the accepted ergonomic principles.

He says,

The sitting position should be a 115 degree angle between front thighs and tummy. Designers of seating who assume that the correct angle would be 90 degrees do not question procedures which were used in basic medical practice. This fallacy of the sitting position being at a 90 degree angle is a throw-back to the days when they were students and worked with a skeleton whilst they studied the bone structure. The skeleton, devoid of muscles and ligaments, would only sit straight on a chair at a 90 degree angle. But once ligaments and muscles cover the bone structure the angle of balancing the body would change to 115 degrees.

Raising his 193 cm (6′ 4″) body – with extremely straight supple spine – from his own chair Dr Middleton produces a sitting wedge that he recommends for good posture and the avoidance of back-related problems, for work at the desktop.

This wedge is made from high density foam rubber which is 6 thick at the back, slanting down to less than 1 cm at the thin end of the wedge.

'Soft on the bum,' he says, 'putting no ridges of pressure on any part of the thighs. If someone sits on a hard or immobile seat with a thick edge, that will put pressure on the thighs which can create a circulatory problem resulting in many people suffering from pins and needles, or numbness, in the legs or feet.'[6]

There are now innumerable medical and scientific papers that demonstrate from their own researches why their authors embrace Mandal's principles of twenty years ago.[7-9] They have been widely adopted throughout Europe, Scandinavia and North America. I can find no British manufacturer who has adopted them, though several manufacturers to whom I spoke have said that they are intending to rectify that position very soon.

Extensive worldwide studies report that the adoption of Mandal's recommended type of seating causes the pelvis to rotate forward, thereby causing the lumbar spine to assume a concave posture, which relieves pressure on lumbar discs. Succinctly, the features required of this medically acclaimed seating call for:

1 A 15 degree forward tilting seat.
2 Adjustable seat height to suit individual heights.
3 A solid base on five legs with castors to provide stability and movement of chair as required.
4 Contoured back rest shaped to support the lumbar region and spine, with adjustable backward tilt to facilitate individual preferences for reclining and relaxing.
5 All to be available in an assortment of sizes – like clothes – to fit the multiplicity of body sizes.

Granjean and his colleagues, whilst agreeing that the 90 degree angle was wrong, argued that proper design of an ergonomic chair should allow the operator to assume a backward leaning posture, with the arms supported by an adjustable chair arm and a wrist/palm rest. This posture automatically provides support to the lower back by maintaining the weight of the trunk against the back rest. Moreover, operators seem to prefer this orientation to being upright.[10]

The operators' choice

Fixtures Furniture Inc. of Kansas City funded an expensive and intensive independent study carried out by the Center for Ergonomic Research at the Department of Psychology at Miami University. They monitored the medical effects, photographed and took video recordings of workers using the different types of chair mechanisms when performing both VDU and non-VDU tasks. They had the choice of forward tilting seats, sitting at the 90 degree angle, backward tilting seats and multiple variation on the tilt of back rests and height. The results were consistent. Preferences were:

1 The seat pan tilted forward 15 degrees when the work was copy intensive. At the end of the test period there were no potential health problems reported with this type of seating.
2 The back rest tilted backwards 15 degrees when the task was screen-intensive.[11]

Kneelers I cannot find anyone to put in a good word for these, which usually have a seat slanting to 45 degrees necessitating the knees to be placed on a pad, encouraging damaging and constant pressure on the very delicate knee structure. They are a recipe for disc problems, painful knees and circulatory problems in the legs.

The consensus of opinion is that kneelers are an exaggerated interpretation of the 15 degree forward tilting seat. They are marketed with the knowledge that many members of the public will try anything if it is new – particularly if they are suffering from a back problem and acquisition promises a cure!

The desk

No operator should ever have to put up with trailing wires and cables or have to crawl under or behind desks to connect sundry electrical items to the power supply. These practices are dangerous and the configuration of wires and plugs that frequently results is already illegal in Britain. Strategically placed electrical sockets at work-top level will cater for personal ionisers, calculators, dictating machines, answerphones and the rest. Virtually all of today's VDU desks have a built-in facility to do this. By the end of 1992 it will be a legal requirement in the EC.[12, 13]

Desk design

Ergonomically designed desks and work terminals for VDUs all have facilities built into them which separate and secure all the different wires that need to be connected variously to 'clean' and 'dirty' power supplies. This is known as *wire management*. An additional important benefit is the prevention of dust accumulation.

The enlightened way (now common practice in what has become known as office landscaping) is to bring power to the work terminal via ducting under a slightly raised false floor. A small piece of carpet is removed at the back of the desk, so that the requisite wires can be brought up to an assortment of neatly cut-out channels which have been built into the frame of the desk.

Desk-top equipment is connected to the appropriate electrical supply by threading the leads through removable access plates situated in strategic points on the work surface. A removable panel on the back of the desk covers the wires, preventing dust collecting and providing an aesthetically pleasing and easily cleanable environment whilst, at the same time, ensuring that there are no trailing wires for operators to trip over.[12, 13]

Alternatively, if the terminal backs on to a wall, the power supply can be directed from that source, provided that the terminal is easily removable for unrestricted access of servicing engineers, replacement or addition to the wiring configuration, cleaning purposes, etc.

If required, further power points can be placed along the top or side of the desk so that occasional additional pieces of equipment can be easily connected. A small calculator, an occasional task light, a personal ioniser or the office vacuum cleaner can be connected to one of these.

The conductivity of the structural materials of the desk is important. A person may get an electric shock if they touch a metal frame because of the static build-up inherent near every VDU. Solid wood provides the most suitable structural material. Front edges should be rounded so that they cannot block circulation in wrists or arms when they are in a resting or handwriting position.

Polished or shiny work-tops are to be avoided. They must have matt surfaces, both to eliminate reflections and glare and to help absorb sound.

Work surfaces for VDUs need to be much wider than the old desks used for typewriters. There must be sufficient depth to accommodate the VDU and its keyboard and allow the operator to rest forearms on the desk in front of the keyboard. That means a minimum of 1000 mm to take a 20 megabyte hard-disk PC.

The type of work will determine the length of the work-top. Adequate provision has to be calculated for all the sundry pieces of equipment to be placed on the work-top, along with the number and size of files and documents which the operator might require during the course of work. It must also have sufficient space around it to allow the operator to move body, work and chair away from the screen when performing non-keyboard tasks.

The minimum size of desk must leave unrestricted leg space under the work-top of not less than 660 mm height and 1200 mm width.[12] Therefore, if drawers or cupboards are required underneath the desk-top, the width of those must be added on to the minimum 1200 mm required for free leg space.

Because floor space is sometimes restricted for economic reasons, some manufacturers are building terminals with cupboards and shelves set at the back of the work-top so they look almost like fitted kitchen units. Apart from the fact that storage on these upper levels reduces the amount of floor space required (the economic logic of the high-rise building) these manufacturers feel that they are making the VDU task easier by putting everything that the operator might need within arm's reach from the desk-bound sitting position.

But is this a good idea? My own view is that it is unwise to restrict physical movements even more – in what is already an unhealthy sedentary occupation. Of course the reduced costs may be a good idea from the employer's point of view; the more equipment and consequently the larger numbers of employees you can cram and cramp into a small space also minimises the costs for lighting, heating, and so on.

It is impossible to standardise work-top height to suit the varying heights of people. Yet many offices do this for aesthetic reasons rather than the health and well-being of the operators.

Since average human height has increased whilst the height of desk-tops has been reduced,[4] it would clearly be uneconomical to expect employers to have a desk tailor-made to the size of every newcomer. The only alternative is that, like most chairs, the height and tilt of the work-top should be adjustable.

The new EC standards call for a minimum height of 720 mm for fixed working surfaces and a range of 650 mm to 850 mm for adjustable surfaces.

It is a long time since most of us saw a tilted work-top – probably not since school days, and today even most school desks have been replaced by the flat tables. Yet medical tests demonstrate that for most non-VDU desk-bound jobs performed in the work terminal a comparatively high work-top with a slanted top affords the most physically beneficial working posture.[1-3]

A word of warning; never use a VDU in overcrowded cramped conditions. Test all the facilities offered in any piece of furniture. Do not be misled that furniture is of a sound design merely because the manufacturer or salesman says it is ergonomically designed. There are some absolutely horrendous trolleys/VDU-tables/work-stations claiming to be 'ergonomically designed'. You will see them illustrated in glossy catalogues and displayed in suppliers' showrooms. They are not designed for the benefit of the VDU user. They are designed to get the maximum amount of equipment, and the operator, into the smallest amount of space.

Some are designed vertically in tiers that even include holders for printer and paper under the work-top, to save office space at the expense of the operators' space. This will adversely affect their health by restricting the essential leg space to which they are entitled under the new laws, increasing noise levels and radiation exposure and introducing adverse conditions for the eyes and poor sitting positions.

I am told that many schools have bought these!

Surgeons assess the best posture for non-screen work

Numerous medically controlled experiments have been performed to determine both the chosen and the physically most beneficial heights and angles for co-ordinating work-tops to chair seats. They have looked at large numbers of people of widely differing heights and weights, whose ages ranged between 7 and 50.

During one such series of tests fifty different photographs were taken at timed intervals of each of the individual subjects. Each person was sitting at a desk performing non-screen work.

Both desks and chairs were based on hydraulic columns so that the seated operator could tilt, raise or lower both chair and table slowly to the position that they preferred. There was also a traverse bar, representing a footstool, whose height could also be altered.

The photographs were used to calculate body movements, together with the angles of hip, back, neck and head.

We all understand the temporary strain involved when we deliberately 'flex our muscles' for a while. Did you realise that our back muscles are unconsciously flexed by varying degrees if we sit in a bad posture? After a prolonged period this will cause quite severe (sometimes irreversible) back problems.

This series of photographs measured the degrees of unconscious flexing that were taking place in the flexor muscles of the backs of the test subjects. In one young woman, flexion of the lumbar region was 42 degrees at a table height of 72 cm; it was 25 degrees at a table height of 82 cm; and it was 10 degrees at a table height of 92 cm. The 17 degree reduction in flexion in the lumbar region when changing from 72 cm to 82 cm table height is very significant. So too is the 15 degree reduction from 82 cm to 92 cm.

The most physically beneficial sitting position for this particular young woman – which gives her a 32 degree reduction of flexion in her lumbar region – means her worktop must be 20 cm higher than the recommended height adopted by CEN and most furniture manufacturers.

In these same tests the flexion in the hip joint was found to be 57 degrees at a table height of 72 cm; 50 degrees at a table height of 82 cm; and 42 degrees at a table height of 92 cm.[15-18]

Figure 22.1 shows people's preferred heights for desks and chairs, compared with the CEN recommendation. It may help you choose the best settings for yourself.

Scott Middleton of the British Chiropractic Association told me;

The slant on the old Dickensian desks, today's architects' drawing boards and the old upwardly slanting shape of old typewriter keyboards all offer a more sound ergonomic design for people, reducing or eliminating muscular skeletal problems. Certainly the muscular skeletal problems of today's office workers were unknown in the past by people working with the now almost obsolete sloping designs.

His views echo those of Mandal.

My design for the basic work-station of the future

The work-top

Office furniture designers need to re-think completely and to take notice of the worker's actual needs rather than the aesthetic, whimsical creation which architects and designers dream up, without any personal experience of working for prolonged hours with a VDU, and without having done sufficient medical research.

1 There is a call for entirely new modular designs, with matt finishes, preferably constructed out of wood but otherwise certainly out of non-conductive materials. Each terminal should include three different types of work-tops, including sloping work-tops at two heights – one for standing and one for sitting – and a flat work-top, whose height is

adjustable at the touch of a button by gas cylinders (like those used in modern chairs). Westinghouse have for some years made work-tops whose height is easily adjustable in millimetres.

2 The work-tops for VDU work should be at least 1000 mm deep from front to back, (which they will have to be to comply with new laws, allowing arm space in front of the keyboard). There is less stress and strain on the torso with an L-shaped return on the work-top, on which to place books and documents that are being referred to during VDU work.

The 'L' return should be able to be placed either at the left or the right side of the VDU, to suit the operator's preferences. Since I am left-handed, I prefer a return on the left side. I find a document holder useful but, like most people using a VDU, there are many occasions when I need to refer to a great many different papers and books and a side-return means that the chair swivels the body round from screen to documents and back without the twists, stretches and contortions that become commonplace if the work surface is one long length.

3 The minimum desk length to be 1650 mm with a minimum working length of 1150 mm on the return.

4 There must be absolutely unrestricted leg space. In most countries the law will require a minimum depth of 1000mm, length of 1200 mm and height of 600 mm.

Cupboards, shelves, drawers and trolleys

These must be bought or designed to fit the type of work and the number of files, directories, books, and other storage, as required. Mobile drawers and trolleys can be pulled out from underneath work-tops or shelving can be placed above and behind the work-top, both for convenience of access to their contents and to give extra work-top space as needed.

None of the storage facilities should be placed underneath the work-top in a way that might possibly interfere with free leg-space in the working area.

Seating

Either one multi-functional swivel chair or two separate ones should be available for every VDU operator. Design features I would like to see built in would include:

1 Adjustable seat height. Unlike chairs of today, it must be capable of accommodating the leg lengths of people who are shorter than 163 cm (5' 4") and taller than 183 cm (6'). Remember that VDUs are being used by most schoolchildren now and nobody markets suitable VDU chairs for them.

2 Seat-pan capable of tilting forward by 15 degrees. The operator could either leave it free to follow the body's movements, or lock it in any one preferred position – for example in a position suitable for static keyboard work, or in the 90 degree resting position when the operator is perhaps leaning backwards – so that the feet remain squarely on the floor.

3 Waterfall front on the seat to prevent pressure on the thighs when the operator is relaxing backwards.
4 Firm but flexible back rest at shoulder blade height, contoured to give lumbar support and supple enough to swivel and tilt with the body, as the person twists, bends or stretches. A 15 to 25 degree backward tilt to recline for relaxation, with the additional facility of being able to lock it in place at one's personal ideal setting for keyboard work. Most of these facilities are already available on the Sensor and Giroflex 44 chairs.
5 Removable and adjustable arm rests.
6 Luxury models could include an automatic massage facility, like those included in medically approved passive exercise tables, to improve circulation and relieve aches and pains during the day!
7 It goes without saying that all of the multi-functional facilities would be controllable by easily reached knobs placed underneath the seat.
8 Seat covers made out of natural fibres.

CHAPTER TWENTY-THREE
Office planning

Entirely new design criteria must be given to offices where hi-tech equipment is to be used.

Space

Each operator's daily routine must be split into VDU work and non-VDU work, so that no more than four hours are spent in any one day near a VDU that is switched on.

If the VDU is not switched off completely, or if other VDUs are switched on in the same room, you are still exposed to the radiation emissions just as much as if you continued working without the requisite rest break. It's rather like the passive smoking syndrome, but worse.

The VDU operator may continue to work at other tasks in the VDU terminal, or move to another location, but either way additional space is needed.

Whilst working at the VDU adequate space must be provided to ensure that the operator's environment is never cramped. There must be space to stand, stretch, bend and enter or leave the VDU terminal area unobstructed.

A realistic detailed list should be drawn up of all the files, papers, telephones, reference books, and other equipment that is, or might be, required for whatever type of work might need to be undertaken in the work terminal. Space should also be allowed for personal belongings such as a brief case or handbag. Then the shape and size of desks, cupboards, drawers and shelving can be determined.

At this stage it is advisable to consider the numbers and types of all the electrical equipment which will be installed and to determine whether power is to be supplied from under the floor or from a wall. This can affect the amount of usable space.

Sufficient space to allow easy access for cleaning and servicing must be left near radiators, behind desks and cupboards etc. This is to facilitate thorough cleaning around, behind and under all the items to prevent the accumulation of dust, mites and micro-organisms. Alternatively, enough space must be provided to move those items of furniture easily if they are mobile.

The position of existing windows and lighting must be assessed to ensure that there is sufficient space to site the VDU terminal where these factors cannot adversely affect the VDU operator.

Not until all these considerations have been taken into account can an appropriate amount of space be calculated.

If the alternative makeshift approach is followed of cramming some VDU equipment, files, telephones and sundry items into an existing small space or office then the operator's health will be at risk. The terminal will not work efficiently. And from the end of 1992 there would be a serious breach of the new EC minimum standards.

Decorations

Because of the nature of the VDU screen it is important that all sources of glare, reflections and bright contrasts of colours are eliminated. Gloss paints and shiny surfaces are taboo in the area of the VDU. Matt, mid-tone pastel shades are recommended by most ergonomists. Walls and ceilings should be painted or covered in materials with a non-reflective matt finish. Furniture and all equipment should have non-reflective matt surfaces.

Floor covering

Avoid all floor coverings that can aggravate static problems. Carpets made wholly of natural fibres are preferable providing they are not tightly fitted from wall to wall and glued down.

If carpets with a synthetic content are laid, they should be regularly treated with antistatic solutions every six weeks or so, depending on use.

Earthed antistatic mats with a carbon content, placed underneath the VDU operator's chair, can solve these static problems. The mat needs to be heavy and large enough to facilitate easy unrestricted movements of feet, vacuum cleaners and chairs so that the edges of the mat do not curl up.

All floor coverings must be vacuumed daily and professionally cleaned regularly to prevent accumulation of dust, dust mites and other health threatening micro-organisms.

Other furniture

The requirement will be different in every office. A realistic assessment of the number and types of books, files and so on must be estimated and appropriate furnishings provided accordingly. The important thing is that each and every piece is easily accessed for cleaning purposes.

Where large open spaces provide distractions from lighting or noise the use of acoustic panels can help to provide a solution – without boxing you in and making you feel isolated.

Great thought must be paid to the noise and radiation levels of additional pieces of hi-tech equipment and only essential ones should be placed near operators. Photocopiers and printers must not be in a room where people are working all day. They should be located in a separate well-ventilated room with external air extraction.

CHAPTER TWENTY-FOUR
Noise

Millions of people become partially or completely deaf due to exposure to hazardous sounds and noise. Noise-induced hearing problems are serious because at the time of the damage people are not aware of any physical injury. Irreversible damage can and does happen during the early stages of exposure.

The growing number of hazardous noises in modern buildings presents a potentially serious problem. People should be aware of how prevalent and harmful noisy work environments are since there is no treatment available for noise-induced hearing loss. Preventative measures are essential.[4]

Measuring noise

The noise frequency range of hearing is from about 20 to 20,000 Hz. The ability to recognise a sound at a respective frequency is known as an 'audiometric threshold', which is recorded in decibels (dBA).

There are sounds both below and above this range which humans generally do not hear. Sound below the audible range is called subsonic or infrasonic. Sound above 20,000 Hz is called ultrasonic.

Normal hearing

Normal, healthy, human hearing can detect even the softest sounds and utterances from a leaf falling against grass to the blast of artillery. Initially it is the ability to hear the softer and less intense sounds that is disrupted in noise-induced hearing loss. If you want to know whether or not your ears are in good condition, try the leaf test – ask a friend to stand behind you in a quiet location and drop a leaf on to grass just behind you. Can you hear it?[5]

When impairment occurs below 3000 Hz the ability to easily understand conversations progressively deteriorates and is often noticeable when people have difficulty in distinguishing some consonants; they can confuse such words as 'fish' and 'fist', 'free' and 'three', and so on. These are the early warning signs that a person's hearing needs to be checked.[5, 6, 8]

Although ageing influences one's ability to hear, its effects are only slight. They don't become apparent until 45 to 50 years of age. Research into age-related hearing reveals poorer hearing for men than for women.[6, 7]

Noise damage

The range of hearing most sensitive to noise damage is between 3,000 and 8,000 Hz. These are frequencies above the range where speech is customarily heard.

Excessive noise damages the intricate structures within the inner ear. Cells, blood vessels, and even the nerve fibres, can be physically damaged as a result of both biochemical change and mechanical disruptions.[6]

Ultrasound

Erratic electrical voltages supplied to the VDU cause vibrating electromagnetic waves in the magnetic core in the flyback transformer, thereby creating a source of ultrasound.

Beneficial effects of ultrasound are used in medical circles for diagnostic and therapeutic purposes, in some navigational equipment, and in the ubiquitous silent dog whistle.

When the sound is at too high a frequency for us to hear, depending on its intensity it can cause damage to the ear because as it vibrates it has the ability to heat human tissue and break up the cell walls.

Medical effects of noise

Medical literature points to many physical conditions whose origins stem from noise.

1 We have all experienced a startled response to sound, such as the screeching brakes of a car or the sudden sound of a fire alarm. Or, we have felt a physical cringe when we have heard chalk screech on a blackboard. We can notice mild to moderate psychological responses. We might physically jump, feel the heart beat faster and so on. Fear reactions may result in releases of catecholamines that can increase the heart rate and raise blood pressure. Although such responses are difficult to measure objectively, it is obvious that people respond differently. Similarly, other noises in both work and recreational activities can contribute to stress-like reaction.

   Noise can affect heart rate or rhythm, increase blood pressure and cause temporary increases in blood cholesterol levels and certain hormones.[9, 10]

2 Long-term effects of exposure to noise can also be associated with cardiovascular and circulatory problems.[11]

3 The World Health Organisation (WHO) summarised a variety of non-auditory phenomena associated with noise and experienced during high levels of noise exposures:[11]

   (a) Interference with sleep and modifications of body functions during sleep.

   (b) Stress-related responses, including adrenal gland secretions, such as epinephrine and norepinephrine.

   (c) Circulatory system responses, such as constriction or dilation of blood vessels and increases in blood pressure.

   (d) Startle responses and reflexes that increase heart rate and blood pressure.

(e) Loss of balance. A person's physical sense of balance is maintained
     primarily by special receptors in the inner ear; when these receptors
     become damaged the person loses his or her sense of balance.

The WHO report also deals with symptoms of nausea, headache,
irritability, reduction in sexual drive, anxiety, nervousness, insomnia,
sleepiness and loss of appetite.[11]

   Noise alone may not be responsible for all these problems, but
nonetheless the WHO says their presence should alert employers and
doctors to consider noise when a patient exhibits such symptoms that are
otherwise not explainable. A loud steady state of noise does have an, often
irreversible, adverse effect on hearing.

4 The Occupational Safety and Health Administration (OSHA) estimates
   that 9.5 million workers in the USA who work or have worked in jobs
   where noise exposures are up to 80 dBA (below the recommended safety
   levels) have been found to suffer from hearing defects. Out of the 28.5
   million people so exposed, 17% suffer mild degrees of hearing loss, 11%
   suffer from material impairment and 5% moderate impairment. That
   represents hearing problems for 33% of those who have been exposed to
   levels *below* the current safety standard.

5 The National Institute for Occupational Safety and Health (NIOSH)
   criteria documents record that damage to hearing occurs at 80 dBA after
   exposure for prolonged periods. Their estimate is that 44% of workers
   suffer from hearing-related health problems. 80 dBA is the level from one
   noisy daisywheel printer.

Health effects of ultrasound

6 Some evidence has linked ultrasonic exposure with fatigue, headaches,
   tinnitus (a continual buzzing, hissing or ringing sound in the ear),
   instability, a feeling of swelling inside the ear, and nausea. These
   symptoms are reported in almost every study of VDU operators.[15-18]

7 In 1984 an American panel of experts warned the National Institute of
   Health that doctors should refrain from using ultrasound imaging during
   pregnancy unless there was an 'accepted medical reason for the
   procedure'. The panel concluded that while ultrasound is a good
   diagnostic tool in risky or complicated pregnancies, they warned that
   there is, as yet, insufficient information to reliably assess the risks of
   ultrasound.[15, 16]

8 Researchers at the Albert Einstein College of Medicine in New York
   found that exposure to diagnostic levels of ultrasound could damage the
   chromosomes of human cells.[17] The results of this study confirmed
   previous findings that ultrasound affects the DNA in animal cells. This is
   still an area of controversy since later experiments performed by other
   scientists failed to confirm this research.[15, 18]

9 An example of progressive noise-induced hearing loss will help us better
   understand the nature of this problem. Table 24.1 shows the effects on a
   worker who spent several years in a noisy office environment. A reference

Table 24.1 Example of the audiometric threshold of a worker who exhibited progressive noise-induced hearing loss[19]

	Frequency (Hz*)											
	Left Ear						Right Ear					
Thresholds* recorded in decibels.	*500*	*1000*	*2000*	*3000*	*4000*	*6000*	*500*	*1000*	*2000*	*3000*	*4000*	*6000*
First reference	5	0	0	10	10	5	0	5	5	10	10	10
1st year	0	0	0	10	10	10	5	5	5	10	15	10
2nd year	5	5	0	10	15	10	0	5	5	15	20	15
3rd year	0	5	5	15	15	15	5	5	5	15	25	10
4th year	5	10	15	15	20	20	0	5	5	20	25	15
5th year	0	5	15	25	30	25	10	10	10	15	25	20
6th year	5	10	20	35	40	30	10	10	15	20	35	25
7th year	0	10	30	45	50	40	15	15	20	30	40	35
8th year	5	15	35	50	55	40	15	20	30	45	55	40
9th year	10	25	40	60	70	50	15	35	45	55	65	50
10th year	10	35	55	70	85	60	20	40	50	65	80	55
11th year	15	40	65	80	95	80	10	45	60	75	90	70

*Frequency is a measure of the pitch of a sound and is expressed in Hertz (Hz). Higher frequencies (4000, 6000 Hz) are usually affected in noise-inducted hearing impairments. Thresholds are recorded in decibels (dB), and the quantities shown under frequency indicate the softest intensity level at which the person could hear the different test tones. (Note: 0 dB is audiometric 'zero', and deviations from optimum normal are recorded in dB hearing levels greater than 0)

audiogram was performed when he began work at 24 years of age. The reference hearing levels revealed normal hearing in both ears across all test frequencies, that is from 500 to 6,000 Hz. (Normal hearing is usually defined as being able to hear decibel levels lower than 25 at each frequency).

By the fourth annual examination, the tests showed a trend of deterioration in hearing, particularly between 3,000 to 6,000 Hz. These early changes in hearing suggest damage due to noise.

Subsequent annual examinations show that the deterioration continued within these higher frequency ranges as well as in the lower range below 3,000 Hz. As the damage involved hearing acuity below 3,000 Hz, the person's ability to hear and understand normal conversations began to be compromised. Therefore this person suffered a significant amount of irreversible hearing impairment within a relatively short span of life before he was 35 years old.

If the OSHA criterion for monitoring hearing ability had been followed (i.e. an average shift of 10 dB or more at 2,000 to 4,000 Hz in either ear from the initial examination) damaged hearing would have been identified during the fifth annual examination. At that point, action could have been taken to prevent further impairment.[19]

Are British safety levels unrealistic?

- *In Britain* the Health and Safety Executive recommends not more than *90 dBA* for continued exposure for *eight hours in any one* day. That level would only be allowed for *two hours per day* by NIOSH. It approximates to working near an underground train all day. APEX (the Association of Professional, Executive, Clerical and Computer Staff) will accept 65 dBA, but stresses that lower levels should be aimed at. The Civil Service Trade Union recommends a maximum of 55 dBA for general clerical work, in any office, with the windows closed. For occupations requiring a high degree of concentration they reduce the level to 50 dBA maximum.
- *In Germany* the legal maximum for noise in any workplace is 70 dBA.
- *In the USA* the recommended maximum level in workplaces is 80 dBA. OSHA explains that the 'action level' (the exposure where one is considered exposed to potentially hazardous noise) begins at 85 dBA for a typical 8-hour day. Allowable durations (minutes or hours of exposure) are reduced by half for ever 5 dBA increase above this limit. For example: 85 dBA for 8 hours per day, 90 dBA for 4 hours per day, 95 dBA for 2 hours per day, up to 115 dBA which corresponds to 7.5 minutes per day. NIOSH reduces these levels to an upper exposure limit of 80 dBA each day. It would permit 80 dBA for an 8-hour day, 85 dBA for a 4-hour day, and 90 dBA for a 2-hour day.

The new EC rules

- The new EC regulations permit 40 dBA for intellectual or conceptual work, 60 dBA in general offices, and 65 or 70 dBA where telephone communications are required. The EC guidelines add; 'Printers, can be very noisy, perhaps even reaching limits set for preventing hearing impairment. They must be shielded with a noise-reducing cover, and, if possible, be placed in locations away from the workstations.'[1-3]

Sources of noise that can damage hearing are kaleidoscopic. Over-exposure to noise must be avoided both on and off the job.[4]

How to protect yourself from noise

Find out the level of noise in your workplace. Professional assessments of noise levels take into account the amount of space, number of people, type of work, and all equipment capable of producing noise. They then assess the degree of noise that people will suffer depending on how far away they are from the source of noise.

It is not unusual for the degree of noise to vary in different parts of large offices. The closer you are to the source of noise (such as whirring fans inside VDUs, the telephone, the printer, etc.) the higher will be your exposure.

Effective control of noise-induced hearing loss is dependent on controlling noise at its source, in the form of engineering controls and other acoustic treatments.

Measures you can take include:

1 Place noisy equipment in a separate room whenever possible.
2 Always use acoustic hoods on printers and other noisy equipment.
3 Noise reflects from shiny surfaces, so matt surfaces will reduce the problem.
4 Sound-absorbing material on walls and ceilings will reduce noise around the VDU terminal.
5 Many modern floor coverings cause sound to reverberate. Carpets laid on good underfelt will absorb noise.
6 In large offices groups of workers can be separated by adding sound-absorbing partitions.
7 Does the level of noise in the general office exceed 70 dBA? For intellectual or conceptual work the noise level must not exceed 40 to 50 dBA.
8 Have your hearing regularly checked. Hearing is not usually a concern of the doctor until the capacity to hear and understand speech has been compromised. On the other hand occupational medicine, as a discipline of preventative medicine, is concerned with recognising early changes before this impairment develops. An industrial hygienist is able to evaluate minor changes which may ultimately affect a person's hearing.

CHAPTER TWENTY-FIVE
Lighting

Screen-based technology and operators' health problems have grown at such a rapid rate that they have largely out-paced the development of suitable lighting systems. Researchers have concluded that poor lighting design is a major factor of several health problems suffered by VDU users.[24-31]

Each operator will need light from two basic sources – background light (general room lighting) and task lighting.

Measuring lighting

Lighting levels can be accurately checked with the use of comparatively uncomplicated light meters. However, even without taking measurements of light sources, the problems can be recognised and remedied quickly and simply because you can see them. Meanwhile let's explain:

The *intensity* of light is measured in *candelas*, the basic unit of light measurement. The intensity of a stearine candle is approximately equal to one candela. One candela emits about 12.5 lumens.

Luminous flux is the radiation from a light source and it is measured in *lumens*.

Illumination is the luminous flux per unit of the surface area and it is measured in *lumens per square metre*. One lux is one lumen per square metre.

Luminance is the light which reaches the eye from an illuminated or self-luminous surface. It is measured in *candelas per square metre*.

The *reflection factor* is a measure of a surface's ability to reflect light. Together with the illumination the reflection factor affects the luminance of a surface. It is usually expressed as a decimal between zero and one, or as a percentage.[1-3]

At the VDU terminal

The VDU operator's work is visually demanding. Eyes must adjust from screen to keyboard to desk-based copy. Lighting must be well positioned, give good contrast, and have the colour balance of natural daylight. All light bulbs and fluorescent tubes must be diffused by suitable shades, and there must be absolutely no perceptible flicker.

The lighting at the terminal comes from four quite different sources: (1) the fluorescent letters on the screen (subject to flicker); (2) background lighting (often fluorescent and subject to flicker); (3) task lighting (frequently fluorescent and subject to flicker); and (4) changing natural daylight from windows.

The recommended levels of lighting are as follows. Background lighting in working areas should be between 150 and 500 lux with glare shielding covering the light source, to safeguard against both direct and reflected glare. In general offices where non-VDU work is carried out the recommended level of lighting is much higher at 750 to 1,600 lux. Desk-based work and screen work are incompatible under the same light source.

Task lighting on the work-top needs to have an adjustable swivel arm. It should be supplied with a dimmer switch so that the light on the work-top can be adjusted to fall within the range of 500 to 800 lux, as required.[4-7] In order to minimise visual fatigue, the luminance ratios between the keyboard and the screen, the desktop and the brightest part of the room as viewed from the operating position should not exceed 1:3:10.[3]

Health problems caused by inadequate lighting conditions

1 Epidemiological studies have found that over 91% of VDU operators suffer from tired or sore eyes, eye strain, stress, headaches, fatigue, nausea and muscular problems. Although these problems are frequently blamed on the VDU they may actually result from inappropriate lighting and badly sited equipment.[8-12, 24-31]

2 When light penetrates the eye, impulses are sent not only to visual areas of the brain but also to other parts of the central nervous system.[9] Several studies show that the amount, quality and colour of light will influence body metabolism and temperature, hormone secretion, ovulation and a variety of other basic functions.[13-15]

3 Other research shows that artificial light is more stressful than natural daylight, increasing the eye's production of melatonin which adversely affects the pineal gland, the hypothalamus and the pituitary gland. The results can lead to certain types of psychiatric disorder such as stress, lethargy and depression.[16-19]

4 Experiments carried out in Sweden in offices supplied with different types of fluorescent lighting (both white and daylight type) analysed the effects on the hormones melatonin and cortisol. They found that under daylight tubes workers suffered far less visual fatigue and felt more energetic; and that the production of melatonin was beneficially suppressed.[20, 21]

5 Another salient finding was that regardless of the type of artificial light, people working close to a window produced more of the anti-stress hormone cortisol in summer than in winter. The reverse was true of people sitting far away from the window.[21, 22] The beneficial production of cortisol reduced stress levels, boosted energy and gave a feeling of general well-being.

6 Observations were made over a period of one year on four groups of schoolchildren working under different lighting conditions. The conclusion was that in rooms without windows hormone production became dependent on artificial lighting that could produce a disturbance or even a partial reversal in the annual biological rhythm.[22]

7 Light and colour affect the central nervous system. This can be measured in terms of the electrical activity of the brain, heart beat or emotional mood. Glaring or flickering light, especially in the long wave range, causes severe activation and stress.[10, 11, 15, 18, 23]

Getting the best lighting

Background light

1 Neither natural light nor artificial light should be reflected either directly or indirectly onto the screen. Reflections can create eye strain, headaches and bad posture resulting in muscular problems. These types of reflections on the VDU screen can also affect the hormones, interfere with sleep patterns and cause stress, lethargy and depression.[13-19]

2 General room lighting should be between 300 and 500 lux and give an overall even light.[4, 6, 7]

3 If ceiling-mounted fluorescent tubes are installed they must be fitted with diffusers or screens to shield the lamp. The operator should be positioned between rather than under these so that the lights are running parallel to the operator's line of vision – and parallel to the line of windows.

4 The appropriate level and design of the lighting should be determined by the nature of the work being done. If an operator is only required to look at the screen, which normally has a dark background, then generally a low ambient room lighting level of 150 to 300 lux is required.[33] Occasionally, an operator may prefer a slightly brighter ambient level of 300 to 500 lux.[27] The US military recommends levels as low as 50 lux for screen-based work.[34]

   If the screen has a light-coloured or white background a higher ambient room light level of 500 to 800 lux can be tolerated.[35]

5 Light bulbs and fluorescent tubes with a spectral quality of daylight should always be installed rather than the traditional cool-white lighting.[8-11]

6 Avoid ceiling-mounted spotlights. They concentrate heat on the back of the neck.

7 Providing that the ceiling is not too low, up-lighting at strategic points is ideal because of its diffused nature.

8 Indirect tungsten light bulbs are frequently recommended because they give a steady forgiving light.[32] These are the common domestic light bulbs.

9 Most fluorescent lights operate at the mains frequency of 50 cycles a second. Even if there is not a perceptible flicker from this type of light the eye and brain subconsciously detect that flicker and it can be an additional source of eye strain and stress.

   50 cycle frequency fluorescent tubes have been responsible for many accidents occurring in industrial workshops. Because the frequency cycle of the fluorescent light can be the same as revolving blades or mechanisms, when the light and the mechanism are synchronised, workers do not detect the movement. Mistakenly assuming the blades are stationary, they reach out to touch, and hands and fingers have been maimed.

   If the employer or school insists on having fluorescent lights in the VDU terminal area, ask for the new high-frequency tubes to be fitted

(28,000 cycles per second). These cost a bit more to install but there are savings on running costs and benefits from noticeably reduced eye strain.

Task lighting

10 Every VDU operator must have a task light on the work-top to provide a controllable spotlight on documents and papers that are required as part of the work being performed.

11 The task light should have a dimmer switch so that the intensity of the light can be controlled as required, in the range of 500 to 800 lux.[4, 35]

12 Regrettably there are a number of futuristic task lights being sold that are totally inappropriate for the purpose which they claim to serve. Some in fact would increase problems. Design characteristics must include:

(a) A light source completely free of flicker. Many task lights use 50 cycle fluorescent tubes that are subject to flicker. On a work-top so close to the operator's eyes that is absolutely unacceptable. Insist either on a tungsten lamp or a high-frequency (28,000 cycles per second) tube.

(b) The light source must be covered with a completely opaque tilt and swivel shade that allows light to be directed on to different shapes and sizes of documents in use alongside the VDU.

(c) The head of the light, its shade and the stem, must be sufficiently adjustable to allow repositioning of the height and angle of the light so that it gives both full illumination of documents of various numbers and sizes on the work surface and at the same time cuts off the light beam completely, where required. This will prevent any light scatter being detectable either on the operator sitting in front of the screen, or on the keyboard or the screen itself.[5]

(d) The base of the light must be heavy enough to stay in place when the light fitting is bent and stretched in different directions.

(e) There must be absolutely no vibrations from any part of the task lamp.

13 Some fluorescent fittings have black mesh strips, of diminishing thickness and pattern, painted around the length and circumference of the tube. The idea is that the fluorescent tube can be rotated by the operator when and as required, to control the contrast and intensity of light on the work surface. These lights are incorporated into modern work stations and are located beneath cupboards and shelves built on at the back of the work-top (similar to contemporary fitted kitchen units).

In most cases the position of the VDU itself, twixt light source and operator, will stop the light reflecting on the screen, keyboard and operator.

However, some of these patterned tubes still use the old style 50 cycles per second tubes and, if so, no matter how diffuse the black lines make the emitted light, the brain and the eye are not deceived. If flicker is present it can be harmful. The fittings must incorporate the new high-frequency tubes operating at 28,000 cycles per second and be balanced to daylight.

Windows

14 In the vicinity of the terminal, windows must be fitted with adjustable blinds so that operators can control the amount of light and brightness near the VDU. There must be absolutely no reflections or glare from windows visible on the screen.

15 If the VDU is near a window it must be positioned at right angles to it. Operators should not sit facing windows because they would be exposed to direct glare.

16 VDU screen must never face a window because that will create problems of shadows, reflections and glare on the screen.

17 It is important that operators have control over ventilation in the work area. They should have the freedom to open and close windows if and when desired, and be able to adjust thermostats on nearby radiators.

CHAPTER TWENTY-SIX
The sick building syndrome

It's an ironic coincidence that during the highly symbolic year of 1992 the Berlaymont building in Brussels, that houses the 3,000-strong elite of the EC bureaucracy, will be demolished because it has become an extremely sick building. It suffers from numerous problems attributable to air-conditioning and ventilation, and from decaying contemporary building materials that are polluting the air with toxic powder.[39] Similarly, visually prestigious buildings belonging to some of the most affluent international organisations are exposing workers to sickness and death.

Since the 1973 oil crisis employers have become over zealous in their efforts to meet the government's directives to conserve energy whilst, at the same time, boosting company profitability by cutting costs of building materials, furnishing, heating and ventilation. They then equip these buildings with radiation emitting VDUs and an assortment of other hi-tech electronic gadgets with the potential to cause severe physical damage to employees.

Contemporary hospitals, shops, offices, schools and hotels mislead us into thinking they are clean, healthy, efficient and prestigious buildings. In fact, most of them are breeding grounds of a range of health hazards. The Orbit study found that 80% of London's leased offices are at least partially inadequate to support office automation.[31] In July 1991 a British all-party Commons committee chaired by Sir Hugh Rossi identified up to 800 toxic vapours in some sick-buildings which Sir Hugh described as unsuitable conditions for millions of office workers – costing British industry £650 million a year in days off.

Old traditionally built buildings afford a far greater degree of safety than modern buildings, while at the same time being suitable for hi-tech equipment – if the introduction of that equipment is planned with due care.

What makes a building sick?

1 *Air-tight double glazed windows* that cannot be opened easily, wide enough and often not at all.
2 Older healthy buildings become 'sick buildings' when *nooks, crannies and chimneys are blocked and sealed* to prevent any exchange of air with the outside.
3 *Doors* are made to swing shut so that the very minimum exchange is made between the air inside and that outside.
4 *False ceilings* have become dust traps and breeding grounds for micro-organisms.
5 *Cavity wall insulation* prevents fresh outdoor air from seeping into and out of the building.
6 *Water cooling towers* installed as part of the heating/cooling system

provide a breeding ground for legionella bugs, other bacteria, fungi and viruses.

7 *Pipes and radiators* are notoriously too close to walls, collecting dust and making thorough cleaning difficult if not impossible.

8 *Air-conditioning pipework and ducting* collect dust and provide a breeding ground for bacteria, fungi and viruses that can be transmitted into the circulating air, if air filters are not checked and replaced and ducting regularly cleaned. At the same time, the same old recycled air can become impregnated with bugs and viruses from assorted sneezes and unhealthy workers, tobacco smoke, body odours, food smells, dust, fibres and volatile chemicals like ozone, PCBs (emitted by some older VDU screens), aldehydes and formaldehyde released from office equipment, CFCs present in chemicals to clean components in computers and VDUs, other cleaning chemicals, and chemicals emitted from furnishings, fittings and construction materials.

9 *Humidification systems* introducing jets of vaporised water into the air system can be another source of infection and sickness if the water storage system and all the component parts – particularly the air ducts which are prone to becoming blocked – are not regularly cleaned and sterilised.

10 *Building materials.* Dr Wilfreid Kreisel, director of the environmental health division of the World Health Organisation, told the World Federation of Building Contractors, meeting in Birmingham in 1990, that during the past 40 years a shortage of porous, traditional and natural building materials, particularly wood, has led to the development of new types of structural building materials that are not porous. They form an impenetrable shield against air movement.

These, along with solvents emitted from fabrics and cleaning agents, artificial fibres, plastics, new cleansers and insecticides with unknown effects on air quality, have become commonplace – progressively polluting the air inside buildings.

Dr Kreisel described air polluted by micro-organisms, as well as volatile chemicals and hazardous fibres, causing skin allergies, chest infections, gastric and eye complaints. He confirmed that the WHO acknowledged the growing incidence of headaches, pains and general discomfort, as unavoidable in air-tight, air-conditioned buildings filled with VDUs and other electronic equipment.[8-24, 28]

11 *Radon gas*, the naturally occurring radioactive gas, leaks from the ground into homes and buildings and may present a risk in some air-tight buildings.

A parliamentary inquiry in the UK is being urged to recommend firmer action to protect thousands of offices and homes from dangerous levels of this cancer-producing gas. *The Times* has reported that lung cancer caused by radon gas kills an estimated 2,500 people a year in Britain.

In America the Environmental Protection Agency estimates that 20,000 deaths a year are caused by exposure to radon gas and Dr Denis

Henshaw, a physicist leading a team from Bristol University in Britain, suspects a leukaemia connection from radon gas because, he says, alpha radiation penetrates bone marrow.

The National Radiological Protection Board admits that high levels of radon are a big public health problem in the UK. The extent of the radon menace in workplaces is still not clear but the Board says that 'it is likely to be appreciable'.[27]

This is a geographical problem depending on the rock formation in different parts of the world. In Britain the areas most affected are Devon and Cornwall, the granite areas found in Somerset, Northamptonshire and Derbyshire and the north of Scotland. They have high radiation levels, sometimes ranging between 400 and 1,000 bequerels per cubic metre. The national average is 20 bequerels.

12 *Electropollution and radiation.* Every piece of electrical equipment and wiring configuration within the building creates a source of various types of radiation, static and electromagnetic fields around it. Also, electrical machines in buildings are constantly discharging harmful positive ions and destroying the beneficial negative ions in the atmosphere.

It has been found that electrical appliances are, in practice, often 'earthed' via the structure of a building rather than through the wire designed for the purpose. These unbalanced earth returns can produce surprisingly high electric fields, especially when metallic materials concentrate the fields. Aluminium-backed plasterboard, ribbed steel joints, and even radiator systems can all cause abnormally high ambient fields.[38]

13 *Fluorescent lighting* is frequently a large contributory source of health problems in sick buildings. Lights generate a considerable amount of heat and interfere with humidity levels. Fluorescents are also a source of PCBs, ultraviolet radiation, ozone and flickering. Like the VDU screen their light source utilises a glass tube coated inside with phosphorus activated by an electrode at each end of the tube which converts electromagnetic radiation into visible light.

Because it is more important to VDU operators than to any other sector of workers, we have dealt with the particular lighting requirement of someone using a VDU in the previous chapter.

When performing non-VDU tasks it is still important that when fluorescent lighting is used, the tubes are covered with diffusion shades and are preferably of the high-frequency type.

14 *Noise and ultrasound* problems are attributed to a wide assortment of machinery and equipment found in most buildings. A general measurement of noise in the centre of a building or office will be quite different from those taken at the exact location of each person in that building or office, depending how close the person is to the source(s) and the tone and pitch of the sound.

Common sources of problems are the component parts of air-conditioning and central heating systems and the cooling fans built into electrical equipment.

15 *Maintenance*. Unfortunately a great deal of suffering is caused because of human neglect, irresponsibility and inefficiency. Whatever the expense or inconvenience, it is vitally important that the interior and exterior of buildings, their furnishings, heating systems, air-conditioning systems and all other equipment are regularly and meticulously cleaned, serviced and maintained.

New equipment must be professionally installed and those who are to operate or maintain such equipment must be trained to do so safely and efficiently.

Buildings and air-conditioning systems belonging to some of the most affluent and prestigious companies have made headline news because equipment, maintenance, servicing and controls have failed to stop outbreaks of legionnaires' disease and humidifier fever. Contaminated water, bacteria in the system and faulty cleaning programmes were all to blame – on some occasions resulting in sickness and death.

Research into causes of sick building syndrome

1 The US Environmental Protection Agency became involved in investigating the sick building syndrome, coinciding with a rather embarrassing problem in its headquarters when chemicals given off by new carpeting made its own staff sick. It embarked on a chemical pollution monitoring programme in other public buildings and found that they frequently contained low levels of common chemicals in the air.

It seemed that these chemical contaminants were slowly being emitted from synthetic materials used to construct and furnish modern buildings. 'They get vaporised,' a spokesman explained, 'and they get trapped in a very small box – the building! They rise to the point where some of us are getting sick.'

Yet these chemicals could only be detected at levels well below accepted safety limits.

There were suggestions that continual exposure to low levels of these everyday compounds might overload people's defence mechanisms, producing symptoms of malaise and lethargy.[26]

2 Only two years after the 1973 oil crisis that heralded the beginning of stringent energy conservation, the first victims were struck. Twenty-nine people died after attending an American Legion convention in a Philadelphia hotel in 1975. Before they died they appeared to have a type of pneumonia, with fever, aches and shivering. Scientists eventually identified a rod-shaped bacterium, contaminating bathroom fittings in the hotel, which they named *Legionella pneumophilia*.[8]

3 In 1985, at Stafford district general hospital in the UK, harmful concentrations of the bacteria carried in a fine spray of water wafted into the atmosphere killing twenty-nine people from legionnaires' disease.[7]

4 In 1984 the Public Records Office at Kew in London was closed for ten weeks after staff working in the £7 million building complained of influenza-like illness. It was not until after £100,000 was spent on

disinfecting the air-conditioning system that the Health and Safety Executive certified the building safe for use.[43]

5 Two men died and dozens were detained in hospital after an infected cooling tower started an outbreak of legionnaires' disease at Broadcasting House in central London in 1988.[40]

6 Five months later, 2,800 workers were sent home from a British Aerospace plant at the end of 1988 after thirty-six workers showed symptoms of legionnaires' disease. Identifying the source of the problem was a formidable operation because of the vast quantities of water which pass through the steam-powered system throughout the plant. Medical scientists from Withington public health department in Manchester had to examine water pipes, central heating ducts, water testing chambers and cooling towers as well as shower units, wash basins and lavatories.[29, 41, 42]

7 At the beginning of 1989 an outbreak of legionnaires' disease in central London killed five people. Amid public panic, whilst efforts were being made to trace the exact location of the cause, sixty-two water towers in forty-two buildings were closed in the Leicester Square area.

Dr Deirdre Cunningham, Westminster Council's chief medical officer, publicly announced; 'We are thinking about scrapping water cooling towers, but we may feel it is appropriate just to scrap the smaller systems. The larger systems have a fairly substantial flow of water through them and do not silt up as quickly as the smaller ones. We feel that there are alternatives for smaller buildings which might be better as well as safer. The recommendations we make would apply to all densely-packed areas of the country.'[29]

8 Sherwood Burge and Tony Pickering, two British chest physicians, investigated mysterious illnesses in a print workshop, claimed to be humidifier fever. Workers developed flu-like symptoms every Monday night, which then progressively abated throughout the week. The cycle was only broken when the humidifier broke down. It was obvious where the cause lay.

The puzzle was that there was nothing particularly pathogenic coming from the humidifier. Burge and Pickering concluded that broken-up particles of normally benign micro-organisms that had been allowed to accumulate in the water reservoirs were being sprayed out into the air and were causing an allergic reaction in the workers.[26]

9 Employers have proved reluctant to allow investigations into their buildings, fearing the expense required to remedy the faults found and the disruption of staff. This is a false economy since staff sickness may erode their profits if their office systems are unhealthy. Rotherham Council's education department at Norfolk House, Rotherham, Yorkshire was an exception. Problems began there shortly after the staff moved into the brand-new building.

Hundreds of people working in that building were having continual unprecedented health problems ranging from skin problems, lethargy, sore throats and snuffles, breathing difficulties and chest problems, to blinding headaches, migraines and eye problems. Even people who only visited Norfolk House for a day found their skin becoming blotchy within just a couple of hours.

Ensuing investigations revealed that 300 from a total of about 600 staff suffered from at least some of these health problems. The symptoms rarely persisted outside the office, and weekends and holidays were usually trouble-free.

Pam Quinn, an employee, explained; 'Whilst the building is cool in the summer, it becomes freezing cold in winter. If someone is smoking on one floor, the people on another floor get it through their air vent the next day.'

In addition to air-conditioning problems, the building was fumigated after investigators found wood beetle in the furniture. And it was discovered that there was a major problem with lighting caused by the lack of natural daylight in many areas and glaring fluorescent lights that continually flickered.

Dr Alex Balsdon commented that since the symptoms suffered are common in any population, it is their timing that points to the diagnosis of the sick building syndrome. Symptoms become worse after the person has been in the building for a few hours and improve when they leave.

Air-conditioned buildings cause more problems than those with natural ventilation. Precise causes are rarely found, but include inadequate ventilation, too high a temperature, too low a level of humidity, poor lighting, lack of negative ions, air-borne dust and fibres, chemical pollutants from cigarette smoke, fabric and furnishings, and micro-biological contamination.[26, 30]

10 Dr Leslie Hawkins, head of the occupational health unit at the Robens Institute at Surrey University, has become a specialist in the sick building syndrome and in electropollution in the VDU environment.

He has seen evidence of a variety of symptoms relating to this problem, ranging from mild to incapacitating, including assorted respiratory difficulties, headaches and eye, nose and throat irritation. He tells me:

The number of things you can become sensitive to in an office is enormous; dead bacteria, moulds, fungi, fibres from fabrics, carpets and paper, tobacco smoke and so on. You have the air brought in from outside which is generally not very clean anyway, and then you add all the indoor stuff and circulate it around. One thinks of the office as being a clean environment, but the air is like a soup of all kinds of things.

The responsible thing to do is to clean up the air wherever possible. Filtration systems must be checked and electrostatic air cleaners fitted. The cost is small in proportion to lost working hours.

It may be that people who are sensitive act as a kind of barometer for the rest of us, indicating through their reactions the presence of a chemical which, in larger doses, would adversely affect us all.

Setting the controls to get the desired effects from recycled air demands detailed knowledge and a precise mathematical assessment which takes into consideration the volume of building space, the number of people occupying that space, the number and types of lighting fittings and all other equipment, and the heat which they generate, the effect the combined heat has on the humidity and the exact nature of gases and chemical pollutants (such as ozone from printers, photocopiers, VDU screens and fluorescent lighting.)

How to make a sick building healthy

1 Photocopiers, laser printers and any other equipment capable of emitting poisonous gases or fumes must be placed in a separate room from the VDU terminal. All such equipment must be fitted with filters which are cleaned and replaced regularly. Extractor fans must be installed to take ozone-laden air out of the building.
2 Natural ventilation systems must be controlled by the VDU operator. These include windows and/or doors that can be opened and shut as required. Mechanical ventilation controlling the actual movement of air must be controllable by the operator. Airflow as low as 0.15 metres per second can be experienced as disturbing. Air velocity should not exceed 0.25 metres per second, with a ventilation rate of 30 to 50 cubic metres of air per person per hour. Ask the boss what yours is![34, 35]
3 Operators should be able to control heating in their own working environment. The temperature should be maintained between 19 and 23 degrees centigrade.[35, 36]
4 Humidity is important both for workers' comfort and to help minimise the static electricity associated with the use of VDUs and other electronic equipment. A humidity of between 40 and 50 per cent is recommended.[35, 37]
5 Ionisers will considerably benefit the health and efficiency of most people.

   Small personal ionisers can be situated on top of the desk. I find a small, inexpensive one alongside and pointing across my keyboard between my body and the screen has made a noticeable difference. However, a word of warning. If the ioniser is not fitted with a filter the 'muck' that it collects will soon be apparent by the dirt on nearby equipment and surfaces. Of course models fitted with filters are more expensive.

   Alternatively, in the case of big offices, larger ionisers can be mounted on walls. Care needs to be taken to ensure that the size and strength of the ioniser is correctly balanced to the size of the area to be treated, the number of people in that space, and the number of pieces of equipment which contribute to the destruction of the natural ideal balance of negative and positive ions.
6 Frequent cleaning, testing and servicing must be carried out on all water tanks, pumps, ducts and pipework used for cooling, heating and adding moisture to the air.

7 Service engineers must perform frequent cleaning of all filters, grills and
   pipework used for ducting and circulating the treated and recycled air.
8 Dust mites and fungal spores can provoke asthma and rhinitis (blocked
   or runny nose caused by allergy). Below 45 per cent relative humidity in
   an ambient air temperature of between 20 and 22 degrees centigrade, few
   dust mites survive. At higher levels mites rapidly multiply up to several
   thousand per gramme of house dust. Regular thorough cleaning is
   necessary, around and behind pipes and radiators, furniture and
   equipment. Daily vacuuming and six-monthly dry cleaning of carpets,
   upholstery, and fabrics will prevent problems from these sources.[25]
9 In the USA, Dr Bill Wolverton from the National Aeronautics and Space
   Administration is researching the beneficial effects plants can have in
   sick buildings. He reports that plants keep the environment healthier by
   absorbing toxic substances in the air. The green spider plant proved
   most effective at getting rid of carbon monoxide; the philodendron at
   absorbing formaldehyde (which is said to cause allergic, flu-like
   reactions) from particle board panelling and carpet backing; and species
   of daisy and chrysanthemum counteract benzene from office solvents
   and some types of felt-tip pen. Sick plants are signs of sick offices![43]
10 Testing for radon gas has been made simple and inexpensive by Dr
   Denis Henshaw of Bristol University and Dr Geoffrey Camplin of
   Portway School. At the beginning of 1990 they launched a do-it-yourself
   radon-testing kit. It's called Tastrak and costs £6. You also need an
   empty cream or yoghurt carton and a small piece of cling film. Here's
   how it works:
   (a) Place a piece of Tastrak in the yoghurt carton, then cover with a
       piece of cling film.
   (b) Dig a hole in the ground (your garden will do) and bury the carton
       in it.
   (c) Wait three weeks – no peeping.
   (d) Retrieve the carton.
   (e) After three weeks the plastic contains microscopic tracks made by
       radiation that can be counted when viewed under a microscope.
       Radiation levels can be ascertained from the changes in the plastic.
   (f) Send the strip back to the laboratory in Bristol for a result.
   This test is being conducted by fifth-formers in 20,000 British schools
   to find out how extensive the radon problems are.
11 Eliminating radon gas in homes and buildings is possible once the
   problem has been identified. Fig 26.1 from the UK Atomic Energy
   Authority shows the measures you can take.
12 Don't use materials likely to create static electricity, such as nylon and
   aluminium, for furnishings or clothing.
13 Don't run air-conditioning systems at a low level. This results in poorer
   air quality.
14 Install wall-mounted electrostatic air filters to reduce airborne pollution.
15 Check that air intakes are not located near hazardous exhaust vents from
   photocopiers, printers etc.

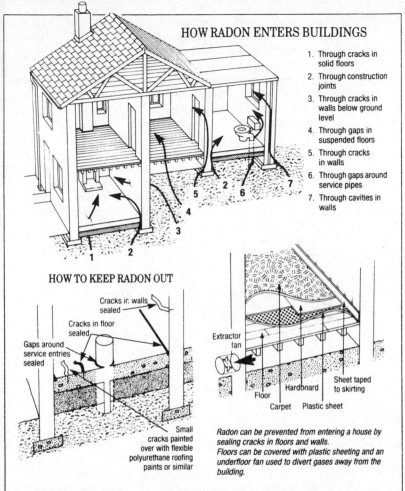

HOW RADON ENTERS BUILDINGS

1. Through cracks in solid floors
2. Through construction joints
3. Through cracks in walls below ground level
4. Through gaps in suspended floors
5. Through cracks in walls
6. Through gaps around service pipes
7. Through cavities in walls

HOW TO KEEP RADON OUT

Cracks in walls sealed

Cracks in floor sealed

Gaps around service entries sealed

Small cracks painted over with flexible polyurethane roofing paints or similar

Extractor fan

Floor   Hardboard   Sheet taped to skirting

Carpet   Plastic sheet

Radon can be prevented from entering a house by sealing cracks in floors and walls.
Floors can be covered with plastic sheeting and an underfloor fan used to divert gases away from the building.

Fig 26.1 How radon enters buildings, and how to keep it out

16 Check that the air quality is monitored regularly.
17 Finally, be aware of the difference between the types of toxic substances that can enter the body – and how they do so. The professionals split them into material and physical agents.

Material agents

The three primary routes of exposure to hazardous materials are inhalation, ingestion and skin contact. Materials can be inhaled if they are present in the form of a gas, a vapour, or an aerosol. The term aerosol refers to dusts (suspensions of finely divided solids in air), mists (droplet clouds), fumes (the condensation or reaction products of a gas), and combinations of these types, such as smokes.

Gases and vapours may be absorbed from the deep lung directly into the bloodstream, may irritate or damage the respiratory tract, or may condense or react with the moisture in the breath to form an aerosol.

Aerosols entering the respiratory tract, or produced there, deposit at locations mainly determined by the size of the particles of the aerosol.[32] The largest tend to deposit in the nose and pharynx. Medium-sized aerosols tend to deposit in the noise, pharynx and bronchi. Fine aerosols deposit throughout the respiratory tract, including the deep lung.

Eating, drinking or smoking in the work area increases the likelihood of ingestion, as does poor personal hygiene. So; don't eat your lunch, smoke or drink in the VDU terminal area or anywhere in a suspect sick building.

Good personal hygiene includes frequent washing of all exposed skin surfaces; finding an uncontaminated area before eating, drinking or smoking; and avoiding transfer of materials to the skin, eyes, nose and mouth from contaminated air and objects.

Physical agents

This group includes high and low relative humidities, sound and vibration, high and low temperatures, radiant energies, and ionising and non-ionising radiations. They affect the body in much the same way as chemical substances.

Many of these agents produce effects similar to those produced by skin contact with material substances. Others, such as ultrasonic and electromagnetic radiation, can penetrate the body to various depths, depending on frequency, and cause damage or heating effects throughout the region of penetration.[33]

These agents have all been dealt with in detail in the earlier chapters, where further guidance will be found.

Warning

If operators feel generally unwell, or particularly if they develop dry or itching eyes, dry or sore throats, headaches, sinus or respiratory problems, nausea, become tired or feel lethargic, develop skin blotches, rashes or spots when in the building, but notice that the symptoms disappear, or feel increased energy and awareness, during time away from the VDU environment, then the control and quality of the air should be professionally investigated.

Meanwhile the most sensible advice is to leave the building until the atmosphere is restored to a condition that makes you feel healthy and alert.

From an isolated retreat on a country hilltop, I conclude this book, sitting at my VDU, in an ancient house built out of wattle and daub and oak beams. Windows and doors are open, a log fire crackles in the background and a yoghurt carton of Tastrak is buried in the herbaceous border.

I reflect on a comment made by Sir John Badenoch, who chaired the first investigation into legionnaires' disease in 1985. He said,

Air conditioning is largely a fashion and is used a good deal more than necessary. People ought to have a pretty shrewd look at whether it would not be better to take in God's fresh air.

References

Part One

Chapters 1-3

1 Wright, P., 'Concern over child X-rays', *The Times*, 6 May 1988.

2 'Bureau evaluates radiation emissions from video display terminals', *Bureau of Radiological Health Bulletin*, 15, 6 (Rockville, Maryland, Department of Health and Human Services, 1981).

3 McKinlay, A.F., *The Results of Measurement of Electromagnetic Emissions from VDUs and a Comparison with Exposure Standards* (Didcot, National Radiological Protection Board).

4 Villforth, J.C., *An Evaluation of Radiation Emissions from Video Display Terminals*, HHS Publication FDA 81-8153 (Rockville, U.S.A., Bureau of Radiological Health).

5 Schiefelbein, S., 'The invisible threat; the stifled story of electric waves', *Saturday Review*, Sept. 1979.

6 Grandjean, E. and E. Vigliani (eds), *Ergonomic Aspects of Video Display Terminals* (London, Taylor and Francis, 1980).

7 *Working with Visual Display Units*, Occupational Safety and Health Series No. 61 (Geneva, International Labour Office, 1989).

8 Hultgren and Knave, 'Discomfort, glare and disturbances from light reflections in an office landscape with CRT display terminals', *Applied Ergonomics*, 5, 1 (1974).

9 'Study by Labour Safety and Hygiene Research Institute of Osaka', *VDT News*, 2 (1984).

10 European Computer Manufacturers' Association, *Ergonomic Recommendations for VDU Workplaces* (March 1984) and *Ergonomics – Requirements for Visual Display Devices* (Final draft Aug. 1985).

11 Zaret, M.M., 'Cataracts following use of cathode ray tube displays', paper presented at the International Symposium of Electromagnetic Waves and Biology, France, 30 June-4 July 1980.

12 German DIN Association, *DIN 66234 Characteristic Values for the Adaptation of Workstations with Fluorescent Screens to Humans*, Parts 1 to 9 (1981).

13 Mikolajzk, H., J. Indulski, et al, 'Effects of T.V. sets' electromagnetic fields on rats' in B. Knave and P.G. Wideback (eds), *Work with Display Units* (Amsterdam, Elsevier, 1987). This book contains selected papers from the International Scientific Conference on Work with Display Units, Stockholm, 12-15 May 1986.

14 Wertheimer, N. and E. Leeper, 'Adult cancer related to electrical wires near homes', *International Journal of Epidemiology*, 11, 4 (1982).

15 Nordstrom, S., E. Birke and L. Gustavsson, 'Reproductive hazards among workers at high voltage substations', *Bioelectromagnetics* (1983).

16 Byrd, E., 'Review of Soviet literature', *Proceedings of the International Forum on Low-level Radiation*, Ottawa, June 1982.

17 *Working to Keep Work Safe*. RIDDOR, Room 414, Health and Safety Executive, St. Hugh's House, Stanley Project, Bootle, Merseyside L20 3QY.

18 HSE 11 (Rev), *Reporting an Injury or a Dangerous Occurrence*, 5/86 M.300. *RIDDOR, The Reporting of Injuries, Diseases and Dangerous Occurrences Regulations* (London, Health and Safety Executive, 1985).

19 HSE 17, *Reporting a Case of Disease. HSE/86 M.200. RIDDOR, The Reporting of Injuries and Diseases and Dangerous Occurrences Regulations 1985* (London, Health and Safety Executive, 1985).

20 Smith, K., *Submissions to the Royal Commission on Matters of Health and Safety Arising from the Use of Asbestos* (Ontario Federation of Labour, 1981).

21 Dyer, C., 'New right to sue on industrial illness', *The Times*, 13 Nov. 1989.

22 M. Barry to author, London, Taylor Woodrow plc., Jan. 1991.

23 Lancranjon, I., et al, 'Gonadic function in workmen with long term exposure to microwaves', *Health Physics*, 29 (1985).

24 Durney, C.H., C.C. Johnson, et al, *Radiofrequency Radiation Dosimetry Handbook*, 2nd ed. (Brooks Air Force Base, School of Aerospace Medicine).

25 Michaelson, S.A., 'Health implications of exposure to radiowave and microwave energies', *British Journal of Industrial Medicine* (1982).

26 Cooper, J., 'My hand injuries have forced me to retire from work', *Best*, 23 March 1990.

27 Adey, W. Ross, 'The cellular environment and signalling through cell membranes', in *Electromagnetic Fields and Neurobehavioural Function* (New York, O'Connor and Lovely, 1988).

Chapter 4: The printer

1 Steen, Christensen, R., 'Ozone emission from laser printers', Incotel press release, June 1990.

2 *Code of Practice for Reducing the Exposure of Employed Persons to Noise* (London, Health and Safety Executive, 1972, rep. 1978).

3 'Health and safety for white collar workers', *FIET Handbook No. 1* (Geneva, International Federation of Commercial, Clerical, Professional and Technical Employees, 1983).

Part Two

Chapter 6: Pregnancy

1 Lee, B.V. and R. McNamee, 'Reproduction and work with visual display units – a pilot study', *Proceedings of the International Meeting to Examine the Allegations of Reproductive Hazards from VDUs, London, November 29-30 1984*.

2 McDonald, A.D., 'Birth defects, spontaneous abortion and work with VDUs', in Knave and Wideback (eds), *op. cit.*

3 Kurppa, K., P.C. Holmberg, et al, *Birth defects, course of pregnancy, and work with video display units* (Institute of Occupational Health, Department of Pathology, University of Helsinki, 1986).

4 Bergqvist, U., 'Pregnancy and VDT work – an evaluation of the state of the art', in Knave and Wideback (eds), *op. cit.*

5 Kurppa, K., P.C. Holmberg, et al, 'Birth defects and video display terminals', *The Lancet* (1984).

6 Westerholm, P. and A. Ericson, 'Pregnancy outcome and VDU-work in a cohort of insurance clerks', in Knave and Wideback (eds), *op. cit.*

7 Bergqvist, U.O.V., article in *Scandinavian Journal of Work, Environment and Health*, 10, suppl. 2 (1984).

8 Denning, J., article in *New Scientist* (1985).

9 Kurppa, J., P.C. Holmberg, et al, article in *Scandinavian Journal of Work, Environment and Health*, 11 (1985).

10 Murray, W.E., C.E. Moss, et al, 'Potential hazards of video display terminals', in DHHS (NIOSH), *Publication No. 81-129* (Washington, U.S. Government Printing Office, 1981).

11 'Pulsed magnetic fields: conflicting results', *Microwave News* (1984).

12 NIOSH Research Report, 'VDT – pregnancy clusters prompt', *Microwave News* (1984).

13 Mikolajczyk, H., J. Indulski, et al, 'Task-load and endocrinological risk for pregnancy in women VDU operators', at study implemented within the project CPBR 11.1.04 coordinated by the Central Institute of Labour Safety, Poland.

14 Gaspard, U., J.M. Foidart, et al, *Ann. d'Endocrinol.* (Paris, 1984).

15 Stuchly, M.A., M.A. Rpacholi, D.W. Lecuyer and R.D. Mann, *Health Physics* (1983).

16 Braidwood, P., 'VDUs: are they safe in pregnancy', *The Sunday Observer*, 7 Aug. 1988.

17 Slesin, L. and M. Zybko, 'Video display terminals – health and safety', *Microwave News* (1983).

18 *Health and Safety at Work*, 6, 4 (London, Civil and Public Services Medical Association, 1984).

19 Sharma, H., *'An investigation of a cluster of adverse pregnancy outcomes and other health related problems among employees working with visual display terminals in the accounting offices at Surrey Memorial Hospital'* (Vancouver, Surrey Memorial Hospital, 1984).

20 Center for Disease Control, 'Cluster of spontaneous abortions', EPI-80-113-2 (Dallas, Public Health Service, 1982).

21 *Study No. 66-32-1359-81: Investigations of Adverse Pregnancy Outcome* (Atlanta, Georgia, Army Environmental Hygiene Agency, 1981).

22 *VDUs, Health and Jobs* (London, LRD Publications, 1985).

23 'Japanese miscarriages blamed on computer terminals', *New Scientist*, 23 May 1985.

24 Ulstein, M., 'Miscarriage disaster link', in *Journal of the Norwegian Medical Association*, Jan./Feb. 1990.

25 Frank, A., *Effects on health following occupational exposure to video display terminals* (Department of Preventative Medicine and Environmental Health, University of Kentucky, 1983).

26 Reported in *VDT News*, 1, 3 (1984).

27 DeMatteo, B., *Terminal Shock. Health Hazards of Video Display Terminals* (Toronto, NC Press, 1986).

28 Jean Seligmann and Pamela Abrahamson in San Francisco and Mary Haggee in Washington. 'Are computer screens safe', *Washington Post* and *VDT News*, July 1988.

29 Reported in *The Morning Star* and *The times*, 29 Aug. 1984.

30 *VDUs and Pregnancy* (London, City Centre, 1985).

31 Vinnikka, David, 'Update: VDUs and pregnancy', *New Technology Bulletin*, (London, The Civil and Public Services Association, 1984).

32 Reported in *The Daily Mail*, 20 Sept. 1984.

33 Fyfe, Gordon, 'Council rapped, tribunal back sacked mum', *Aberdeen Press and Journal*, 22 Sept. 1984.

34 Schnorr, Teresa M., et al., 'Video Display Terminals and the risk of Spontaneous Abortion', *New England Journal of Medicine*, Part 324 (2), 1991.

Chapter 7: Eye troubles

1 Zaret, M., *Statements for hearings of subcommittee on investigations and oversight*, Committee on Science and Technology, U.S. House of Representatives, 12 May 1981.

2 DeMatteo, *op. cit.*

3 Panel report on 'Impact of video viewing on vision of workers', *Work and Vision* (Washington D.C., National Academy Press).

4 Huws, U., *VDU Hazards Handbook* (London, London Hazards Centre Trust, 1987).

5 'EEC Council Directive on the minimum safety and health requirements for work with display screen equipment (Fifth Individual Directive within the meeting of Article 16 (1) of Directive 87/391/EEC) 90/270/EEC', *Official Journal of the European Communities*, L.156/14, 29 May 1990.

6 *Working with Visual Display Units*, Occupational Safety and Health Series No. 61 (Geneva, International Labour Office, 1989).

7 *New Technology: A Health and Safety Report* (London and Home Counties Area Technology Sub-Committee, APEX, 1985).

8 Meyer, J.J., P. Rey, J.C. Schira and A. Bousquet, 'Sensitivity to light and visual strain in VDT operators: Basic data for the design of work stations', in Knave and Wideback (eds), *op. cit.*

9 Wildberger, H. and Z. Arbeit, *Untersuchung in einer Grossdruckerei* Lin. Mbl., Augenheilk 180, (1982), pp 367-9.

10 Rey, P. and J.J. Meyer, 'Visual impairments and their objective correlates', in E. Grandjean and E. Vigliani (eds), *Ergonomic Aspects of Visual Display Terminals* (London, Taylor and Francis, 1980).

11 Meyer, J.J., A. Bousquet, P. Rey and J. Pittard, 'Two new visual tests to define the visual requirements of VDU operators', in E. Grandjean and E. Vigliani (eds), *Ergonomics and Health in Modern Offices* (London, Taylor and Francis, 1984).

12 Ostberg, O., 'Accommodation and visual fatigue in display work', in Grandjean and Vigliani (eds), *Ergonomic Aspects*.

13 Cakir, A., D.J. Hart and T.F.M. Stewart, *Visual Display Terminals* (Chichester, John Wiley, 1979).

14 Woo, G.C., G. Stron, E. Irving and B. Ing, 'Are there subtle changes in vision after use of VDTs?', in Knave and Wideback (eds), *op. cit.*

15 Rubino, G.F., G. Maina, et al, 'Visual impairment and subjective ocular symptomatology in VDT operators', in Knave and Wideback (eds), *op. cit.*

16 Bergqvist, V.G., in *Scandinavian Journal of Work, Environment and Health*, 10, suppl. 2 (1984).

17 Anfossi, D.G., F.M. Grignolo, G. Maina and C. Romano, in *Giornale Italiano di Oftalmologia Occupazionale*, 1, 1 (1983).

18 Boles, Carenini B., G.F. Rubnino, F.M. Frignolo and G. Maina, 'Visual fitness for VDU operators', in Grandjean and Vigliani (eds), *Ergonomics and Health*.

19 Palm, B., *Work Distance and Optical Correction* (Stockholm, Vision Information Council).

20 *VDUs and You* (London, The Association of Optical Practitioners).

21 Zaret, M., 'Cataracts and visual display units', in B.G. Pearce (ed), *Health Hazards of VDTs?* (London, John Wiley, 1984).

Chapter 8: Skin complaints

1 Wedberg, W.C., *Facial particle exposure in the VDU environment: the role of static electricity* (Fantoft/Bergen, Michelsens Institute).

2 Tjonn, H.H., 'Report of facial rashes among VDU operators in Norway', in Pearce (ed), *op. cit.*

3 Olsen, W.C., *Report from the Christian Michelsens Institute, Ref. CMI No. 803604* (Bergen, Christian Michelsens Institute).

4 Sharma, Hari, *op. cit.*

5 Feldman, R.L., *et al*, 'Terminal illness', *Annals of the American Academy of Dermatology*, Feb. 1985.

6 Linden, C. and J.E. Wahlberg, in *Scandinavian Journal of Work, Environment and Health*, 11 (1985).

7 Wahlberg, J.E. and C. Linden, *VDU work and the skin* (Stockholm, National Board of Occupational Safety and Health, 1986).

8 Stenberg, B., *A rosacea-like skin rash in VDU operators* (Department of Dermatology, University of Umea, 1986).

9 Olse, W.C., 'Facial particle exposure in the VDT environment: the rise of static electricity', *VDT News*, 111, 4 (1986).

10 DeMatteo, *op. cit.*

11 Digernes, V. and E.G. Astrup, 'Are datascreen terminals a source of increased PCB concentrations in the working atmosphere?', International Archives of *Occupational Environmental Health* (1982).

12 Slesin, L. and M. Zybko, 'Video display terminals: health and safety', *Microwave News* (1983).

13 Jenson, A.A., 'Melanoma, fluorescent lights and polychlorinated biphenyls', *The Lancet*, Oct. 1982.

Chapter 9: Back problems and other musculoskeletal disorders

1 DHSS certified figures on backache. Supplied by the Back Pain Association, London, Nov. 1990.

2 Kilbom, A., 'Short and long-term effects of extreme physical inactivity', in Knave and Wideback (eds), *op. cit.*3 Greenleaf, J.E. and S. Kozoloswki, *Exercise and Sports Science Review*, ed J. Terjung (Philadelphia, Franklin Inst. Press, 1982).

3 Greenleaf, J.E. and S. Kozlowski, *Exercise and Sports Sciences Review*, ed. J. Terjung (Philadelphia, Franklin Inst. Press, 1982).

4 Greenleaf, J.E.M. in *Journal of Applied Physiol.*, 57, 3 (1984).

5 Rodahl, K., N.C. Birkhead, et al, *Nutrition and Physical Activity* (Stockholm, Almqvist and Wiksell).

6 Vallbona, C., F.B. Vogt, et al, *NASA Contractor Report. NASA CR-71* (Washington, NASA).

7 Hansson, T., 'The back during prolonged sitting', in Knave and Wideback (eds), *op. cit.*

8 Astrand, P.O. and K. Rodahl, *Textbook of Work Physiology*, 3rd ed. (New York, McGraw-Hill, 1986).

9 *Habitual Physical Activity and Health*, Regional Publications European Series No. 6 (Copenhagen, World Health Organisation, 1978).

10 Astrand, I. and A. Kilbom, in *Aerospace Med.*, 40.

11 Bengner, U. and O. Johnell, in *Acta Orthop. Scand.*, 56.

12 Johnell, O., B. Nilsson, K. Obrank and I. Sernbo, in *Acta Orthop. Scand.*, 55 (1984).

13 Nilsson, B.E. and N.E. Westlin, *Clin. Orthop.*, 77 (1971).

14 Garabrant, P.H., J.M. Peters and T.M. Mack, *American Journal of Epidemiol.*, 119.

15 Gerhardsson, M., *Larkartidn*, 83 (1986).

16 Vallbona, C., F.B. Vogt, et al, *NASA Contractor Report. NASA CR-171* (1965).

17 Winkel, J., 'The significance of physical activity in sedentary work', in Knave and Wideback (eds), *op. cit.*

18 Adams, M.A. and W.V. Hutton, in *Spine*, 8 (1983).

19 Winkel, J. and K. Jorgensen, in *Ergonomics*, 29 (1986).

20 Winkel, J. and K. Jorgensen, in *Eur. J. Appl. Physiol.*, 55 (1986).

21 Winkel, J., 'An ergonomic evaluation of food complaints among waiters as a basis for job design', in K. Noro (ed), *IEA '82 The 8th Congress of the International Ergonomics Association* (Japan, Inter Group, 1982).

22 Winkel, J., 'Foot swelling during prolonged sedentary work and the significance of leg activity', in his thesis, *Arbete och Halsa* (Stockholm, Karolinska Institute, 1985).

23 Shvartz, E., J.G. Gaume, et al, in *Aviat. Space Environ. Med.*, 53 (1982a).

24 Shvartz, E., R.C. Reibold, et al, *Aviat Spat Environ. Med.*, 53 (1982b).

25 Winker, J., 'The significance of physical activity in sedentary work', in Knave and Wideback (eds), *op. cit.*

26 Kelsey, J.L., 'An epidemiological study of the relationship between occupations and acute herniated lumbar intervertebral discs', *International Journal of Epidemiology*, 4.

27 Kelsey, J.L. and R.J. Hardy, 'Driving motor vehicles as a risk factor for acute herniated lumbar intervertebral disc', *Am. J. Epid.*, 102 (1975).

28 Frymoyer, J.W., M.H. Pope, et al, 'Epidemiological studies of low back pain', paper presented at the 6th Annual Meeting ISSLS in Göteborg, Sweden.

29 Hansson, T., B. Roos and A. Nachemson, 'The bone mineral content and ultimate compressive strength in lumbar vertebrae', *Spine*, 1.

30 Hansson, T., *The back during prolonged sitting* (Dept. of Orthopaedic Surgery, University of Göteborg, 1986).

31 Riggs, B.L., H.W. Wahner, et al, 'Differential changes in bone mineral density of the appendicular and axial skeleton with aging', *J. Clin. Invest.*, 67.

32 Lindquist, O., C. Bengtsson, et al, 'Changes in the bone mineral content of the axial skeleton in relation to aging and the menopause', *Scan. J. Clin. Lab. Invest.*, 43 (1983) Results from a longitudinal population study of women in Gothenburg.

33 Hansson, T. and B. Roos, 'The changes with age in the bone mineral of the lumbar spine in normal women', *Calcif Tissue Int.*, 38 (1986).

34 Holm, S. and A. Nachemson, *Nutrition of the intervertebral disc. Acute effects of cigarette smoking. An experimental animal study* (Sydney, ISSLS, 1985).

35 Huws, U. and F. Griffiths, *Keying into Careers* (Greater London Council Equal Opportunities Group, 1985).

36 George Teeling-Smith, Office of Health Economics, London, March, 1991.

37 Nuttall, Nick, 'Hi-tech hits the shirkers where it hurts', *The Times*, 21 March 1991.

Chapter 10: Repetitive strain injuries

1 'Journalism Research Report', *View Update*, 1, 3, (Videotex Industry Association, Jan. 1985); and *Mandalink Media*, 26 Feb. 1985.

2 *Guidelines for the Prevention of Repetitive Strain Injury* (Australian Council of Trade Unions, Occupational Health and Safety Unit).

3 Ackroyd, S., *RSI At British Telecom* (British Telecom Data Processing Executive, 1983).

4 Moore, M., *Telecom hit by repetitive strain injury* (West Australian Telecom).

5 Smith, M.J., *Potential Health Hazards of Video Display Terminals* (National Institute of Occupational Safety and Health, 1981).

6 Vetter, H., *Health hazards associated with the use of video display units* (University of Vienna, 1987).

7 *RSI constitutes a real problem* (London, National Union of Journalists, 1990).

8 *VDU Guidelines* (London, SOGAT).

9 Brammer, Gabriele, 'Musculoskeletal disorders at work', paper presented at the international conference, Guildford, University of Surrey, 13-15 April 1987.

10 Brammer, Gabriele, 'VDUs and health', *Health and Safety at Work* (London, Anbar Tear Sheet Library KB47., 1987).

11 'EEC Council Directive on the minimum safety and health requirements for work with display screen equipment (Fifth Individual Directive within the meaning of Article 16 (1) of Directive 87/391/EEC) 90/270/EEC', *Official Journal of the European Communities*, L.156/14, 29 May 1990.

12 *Working with Visual Display Units*, Occupational Safety and Health Series No. 61 (Geneva, International Labour Office, 1989).

13 'Regenerate', *The Times*, 29 March 1990.

Part Three

Chapters 11-18

1 Suess, Michael, J., 'Health impact with video display terminals', in Knave and Wideback (eds), *op. cit.*

2 Linden, V. and S. Rolfsen, 'Video computer terminals and occupational dermatitis', *Scandinavian Journal of Work, Environment and Health*, 7 (1981).

3 Harvey, S.M., 'Electric-field exposure of persons using video display units', *Bioelectromagnetics*, 5 (1984).

4 'Characterization of electric and magnetic fields', *Video Display Units, Report No. 82-528-K* (Ontario Hydro Research Division, 1984).

5 Bergqvist, U.O.V., 'Video display terminals', *Scandinavian Journal of Work, Environment and Health*, 10, suppl. 2 (1984).

6 Grivet, P., *Electron optics*, 2nd ed. (London, Pergamon Press).

7 Olsen, Cato W., *Electric field enhanced aerosol exposure in visual display unit environments* (Bergen, Chr. Michelsen Institute, CMI 803604-1).

8 Cakir, A., D.J. Hart and T.F.M. Stewart, *Visual Display Terminals* (Darmstadt, Inca-Fiej Research Association).

9 Olsen, Cato W., *Science News*, 120, 10.

10 Wallach, Charles, 'Effects of cathode ray displays on human health', paper presented at the Fourth Annual Meeting of the Bioelectromagnetic Society, Los Angeles, California, June 1982.

11 Krueger, Albert, et al, 'Small air ions: their effect in blood levels of serotonin in terms of modern physical therapy', *International Journal of Biometeorology* (1968).

12 Tjonn, H.H., *Report of facial rashes among VDU operators in Norway*, Husat Research Group, Dec. 1980.

13 Rycroft, R. and C. Calnan, *Facial rashes among visual display unit operators*, Husat Research Group, Dec. 1980.

14 Marha, Karel, 'Very low frequency fields near VDUs: an example of their removal', Document No. 0190n (Hamilton, Ontario, Canadian Centre for Occupational Health and Safety).

15 Nylen, P., U. Bergqvist, R. Wibom and B. Knave, 'Physical and chemical environment at VDT work stations', *Proceedings of the 3rd International Conference on Indoor Air Quality and Climate*, vol. 3 (Stockholm, Swedish Council for Building Research, 1984).

16 Michael J. Suess, Denmark, Regional Officer for Environmental Health Hazards, WHO Office for Europe, 1986.

17 National Radiological Protection Board, *Advice on Acceptable Limits of Exposure to Nuclear Magnetic Resonance Clinical Imaging*, NRPB.ASP5 (London, HMSO, 1984).

18 Malanin, G.I., W.D. Gregory, et al, 'Evidence of morphological and physiological transformation of mammalian cells by strong magnetic fields', *Science*, 194 (1976).

19 Nahas, G.G., H. Boccalon, P. Berryer and B. Wagner, 'Effects in rodents of a 1-month exposure to magnetic fields, (200-1200 gauss)', *Aviat. Space Environ. Med.*, 46 (1975).

20 Cook, E.S., J.C. Fardon and L.G. Nutini, 'Effects of magnetic fields on cellular respiration', in M.F. Barnothy (ed), *Biological Effects on Magnetic Fields*, vol. 2 (New York, Plenum Press).

21 Fardon, J.C., S.M.E. Poydock and G. Basulto, 'Effect of magnetic fields on the respiration of malignant embryonic and adult tissues', *Nature*, 211 (1966).

22 Barnothy, M.F. (ed), 'Haematological changes in mice', in *Biological Effects of Magnetic Fields*, vol. 1 New York, Plenum Press.

23 Toroptsev, I.V., G.P. Gargeneyev, T.I. Gorshenina and N.L. Teplyakova, 'Pathologo-anatomic characteristics of changes in experimental animals under the influence of magnetic fields', in Kholodow Yua, (ed), *Influence of Magnetic fields on Biological Objects*, trans. Joint Publications Research Service, JPRS-63038 (Moscow, 1974).

24 De Lorge, J., 'Effect of magnetic fields on behaviour in non-human primates', in T.S. Tenforde (ed), *Magnetic Field Effect on Biological Systems* (New York, Plenum Press, 1979). Proceedings of the biomagnetic effects workshop held at Lawrence Berkeley Laboratory, University of California.

25 Beischer, D.E. and J.C. Knepton Jr., 'Influence of strong magnetic fields on the electrocardiogram of squirrel monkeys (Samiri sciureus)', *Aerospace Med.*, 35 (1964).

26 Beischer, D.E., 'Human tolerance to magnetic fields', *Astronautics*, 7 (1962).

27 Vyalov, A.M., 'Magnetic fields as a factor in the industrial environment', Vestn., *Akad. Med.*, Nuak SSSR, 8 (1967).

28 Beicher, D.E., and V.R. Reno, 'Magnetic fields and man: where do we stand today?', AGARD, *Special Biophysical Problems in Aerospace Medicine*, Part 3, Presented London 1971, *NASA-CR-127049*), and, *Advisory Group for Aerospace Research and Development*, Paris, 1972.

29 Vylaov, A.M., 'Clinico-hygienic and experimental data on the effects of occupational exposure to steady magnetic fields', *American Industrial Hygiene Association Journal*, 43 (1982).

30 McKinlay, A.F., *The results of measurements of electromagnetic emissions from VDUs and a comparison with exposure standards* (Didcot, National Radiological Protection Board).

31 Saunders, R.D. and H. Smith, 'Safety aspects of NMR clinical imaging', *British Medical Bulletin*, 40, 2 (1984).

32 Lee, W.R., 'Little shocks', *Practice of Medicine*, 225 (1981).

33 Cusack, J.A., *Modern Textiles* (1972).

34 Wallach, *op. cit.*

35 Krueger, Albert, et al, 'Small air ions: their effect in blood levels of serotonin in terms of modern physical therapy', *International Journal of Biometeorology* (1968).

36 Tjonn, H.H., 'Report of facial rashes among VDU operators in Norway', Husat Research Group, Dec. 1980.

37 Rycroft, R. and C. Calnan, 'Facial rashes among visual display unit operators', Husat Research Group, Dec. 1980.

38 DeMatteo, *op. cit.*

39 Sulman, F.G., 'The role of serotonin in gynaecology and obstetrics', *The Hebrew Pharmicist*, 14.

40 R. Gualterotti, The Carlo Elba Foundation, Milan. Quoted in F. Soyka and A. Edmonds, *The Ion Effect* (London, Bantam Books).

41 Pearce (ed), *op. cit.*
42 Lee, W.R., 'Working with VDUs', *British Medical Journal*, 219 (1985).
43 Linden, C. and J.E. Wahlberg, 'Does VDT work provoke rosacea?', *Contract Dermatitis*, 13 (1985).
44 Knave, B.G., R.I. Wibom, et al, 'A technical and medical appraisal of the state of the art', *Scandinavian Journal of Work, Environment and Health*, 10, suppl. 2 (1984).
45 Stellman, J.M. and M.S. Henifin, *Office Work Can Be Dangerous to your Health* (New York, Pantheon, 1983).
46 Gale, A. and Christie Brue, *Psychophysiology and the Electronic Workplace* (London, John Wiley, 1987).
47 Pearce (ed), *op. cit.*
48 Grandjean E. and E. Vigliani (eds), *Ergonomics and Health in Modern Offices* (London, Taylor and Francis, 1984).
49 Moss, C.E., W.E. Murray, et al, 'A report on electromagnetic radiation surveys of video display terminals', *National Institute of Occupational Safety and Health DEW (NIOSH) Publication No. 78-129* (Cincinnati, 1977).
50 Weiss, M.M. and R.C. Petersen, 'Electromagnetic radiation emitted from video computer terminals', *American Industrial Hygiene Association Journal*, 40 (1979).
51 Cox, E.A., 'Radiation emissions from visual display units', paper presented at a one day conference on Health Hazards of VDUs, Loughborough University of Technology, HUSAT, 1980.
52 Wolbarsht, M.L., F.A. O'Foghludha, et al, 'Electromagnetic emissions from visual display units: a non-hazard', *Proceedings of SPIE*, 229 (1980).
53 Villforth, J.C., 'An evaluation of radiation emissions from video display terminals', *Bureau of Radiological Health (BRH) HHS Publication FDA 81-8153* (Rockville, Maryland, 1981).
54 United Kingdom Atomic Energy Authority, *Radiation Around Us* (London, Stanford Press, 1989).
55 *Evaluation of Radiation Emissions from Video Display Terminals*, Bureau of Radiological Health Bulletin 20857 (Rockville, Maryland, US Department of Health and Human Services, 1982).
56 *An Evaluation of Radiation Emissions from Video Display Terminals (FDA 81-8153)*, Division of Compliance Stock No. 017-015-00187-3 (Washington, D.C., US Government Printing Office).
57 Bertell, Rosalie, 'The health hazards of video display terminals', *Environmental Health Review*, 26, 1 (1982).
58 *Environmental Health Criteria 16. Radio Frequency and Microwaves* (Geneva, World Health Organization, 1981).
59 Stewart, Alice, 'Radiation dose effect in relation to obstetric X-rays and childhood cancers', *The Lancet* (1970).
60 DeMatteo, *op. cit.*
61 Harvey, S.M., 'Electric field exposure of persons using video display terminals', *Bioelectromagnetics*, 5, 1 (1984).
62 Goffman, John, *Radiation and Human Health* (Sierra Books, 1981).
63 NRPB chart in *The Effects and Control of Radiation* (London, U.K.A.E.A., 19888).
64 Saunders, P.A.H., *The Effects and Control of Radiaton*, 2nd ed. (Harwell, U.K.A.E.A., 1986).
65 *Environmental Health Criteria 16. Radio Frequency and Microwaves* (Geneva, World Health Organization, 1981), pp 96, 97.
66 *Ibid*, p. 101.
67 'USSR – Standards revised at frequency range 300 MHz-300GHz and 50MHz-300MHz', *Microwave News* (1982).

68 Moss, C.E., W.E. Murray, et al, 'A report on electromagnetic radiation surveys of video display terminals', *DHEW (NIOSH) Publication No. 78-129* (Cincinnati, National Institute for Occupational Safety and Health, 1977).

69 Guy, Arthur, 'Health assessment of radio frequency electromagnetic field emitted by video display terminals', a report to IBM office of the Director of Health and Safety, Corporate Headquarters, 1984.

70 Fox, Barry, 'Safety body may strengthen ozone controls for offices', *New Scientist*, 7 April 1990.

71 Hawkins, L.H., 'The possible benefit of negative-ion generators', in Pearce (ed), *op. cit.*

72 Soyka, F. and A. Edmonds, *The Ion Effect* (Bantam Books).

73 Zuk, W.M., M.A. Stuchly, P. Dvorak and Y. Deslauriers, *Investigation of Radiation Emissions from Video Display Terminals* (Ottawa, Radiation Protection Bureau of Health and Welfare).

74 Bergqvist, Ulf O.V., 'Video display terminals and health. A technical and medical appraisal of the state of the art', *Scandinavian Journal of Work, Environment and Health*, 10, suppl. 2 (1984).

75 *BS415 Specification for Safety Requirements for Mains Operated Electronic and Related Apparatus for Household and Similar General Use* (London, British Standards Institution, 1979).

76 Aitken, J.H. and C.R. Hirning, 'Cathode-ray tube X-ray emission standards for video display terminals', *Health Physics*, 43, 5 (1982).

77 Health and Safety Executive, *Visual Display Units: Guidance Notes* (London, HMSO, 1983).

78 National Radiological Protection Board, *Protection against U.V. Radiation in the Workplace*.

79 Cakir, A., D.J. Hart and T.F.M. Stewart, *Visual Display Terminals* (New York, John Wiley).

80 *British Standards Institution (1983) BS4803 'Radiation safety of laser products and systems' Pts 1, 2 and 3* (London, British Standards Institute).

81 American Conference of Governmental Industrial Hygienists, *Threshold Limit Values and Biological Exposure Indices for 1986-87* (Cincinnati, ACGIH, 1986).

82 *Ibid.*

83 Zaret, Milton M., *Cataracts and visual display units* (Scarsdale, N.Y., Zaret Foundation).

84 American Conference of Governmental Industrial Hygienists, *Threshold Limit Values and Biological Exposure Indices for 1986-87* (Cincinnati, ACGHI, 1986).

85 McKinlay, A.F., *The results of measurements of electromagnetic emissions from VDUs and a comparison of European standards* (Chilton, National Radiological Protection Board).

86 Suess, M.J., 'Health impact of work with visual display terminals', in Knave and Wideback (eds), *op. cit.*

87 Cakir, A., D.J. Hart and T.F.M. Stewart, *Visual Display Terminals* (Toronto, John Wiley, 1980).

88 DeMatteo, *op. cit.*

89 Zaret, Milton, 'Statement for hearings of subcommittee on Investigations and Oversight' (Committee on Science and Technology, U.S. House of Representatives, 1981).

90 *Visual Display Units Guidance Notes* (London, Health and Safety Executive, 1983).

91 *Radiofrequency and Microwaves. Environmental Health Criteria 16* (Geneva, World Health Organization, 1981).

92 Bergqvist, Ulf O.V., 'Video display terminals and health – A technical and medical appraisal of the start of the art', *Knave and Wideback (eds)*,, 10, suppl. 2 (1984).

93 Harvey, S.M., *Characteristics of Low Frequency Electrostatic and Electromagnetic Fields, Produced by Video Display Terminals*, report 82-528-K (Toronto, Ontario Hydro Research Division, 1982).

94 Paulsson, L.E., I. Kristiansson and I. Malmstrom, *Staining fran dataskamrar, arbetsdokument a 84-08* (Stockholm, Statens Stralskyddsinsitut, 1984).

95 Weiss, M.M., 'The video display terminals – is there a radiation hazard?', *J. Occup. Med.*, 25 (1983).

96 *Stalning fran dataskamrar* (Stockholm, Straiskyddsinstitut, 1984).

97 *Advice on the Protection of Workers and Members of the Public from Possible Hazards of Electric and Magnetic Fields with Frequencies below 300 GHz: A Consultative Document* (Chilton, National Radiological Protection Board).

98 DeMatteo, *op. cit.*

99 Brodeur, Paul, *The Zapping of America* (W.W. Norton, 1977).

100 'USSR standards have been revised at frequency range 300 MHz-300 GHz and 50 MHz-300 MHz.' *Microwave News* (1982).

101 Dodge, C.H. and Z.R. Glaser, 'Trends in non-ionizing electromagnetic radiation bio-effects research and related occupational health aspects', *Journal of Microwave Power*, 12, 4 (1977).

102 Sigler, A.T., A.M. Liberfield, B.H. Cohens and J.E. Westlake, 'Radiation exposure in parents of children with mongolism (Down's Syndrome)', *Bulletin of the Johns Hopkins Hospital*, 117.

103 McKinlay, A.F., *The Results of measurements of electromagnetic emissions from VDUs and a comparison with European standards* (Chilton, National Radiological Protection Board).

104 Bureau of Radiological Health, *An Evaluation of Radiation Emission from Video Display Terminals*, HHS Publication FDA 81-8153 (Rockville, Maryland, 1981).

105 Bereznitskaya, A.N. and I.M. Kazbekov, 'Studies on the reproduction and testicular microstructure of mice exposed to microwaves', in Z.V. Gordon (ed), *Biological Effects of Radiofrequency Electromagnetic Fields* (Arlington, Virginia, Joint Publication Research Service No. 63321).

106 *Biological Effects and Health Hazards of Microwave Radiation*, Proceedings of an International Symposium, Warsaw, 15-18 October 1973 (Warsaw, Polish Medical Publishers, 1974).

107 Pearce (ed), *op. cit.*

108 Lancranjon, I., et al, 'Gonadic function in workmen with long term exposure to microwaves', *Health Physics*, 29 (1985).

109 *Ibid.*

110 Brodeur, Paul, *The Zapping of America* (W.W. Norton, 1977).

111 Dodge, C.H. and Z.R. Glaser, 'Trends in non-ionizing electromagnetic radiation bio-effects research and related occupational health aspects', *Journal of Microwave Power*, 12, 4 (1977).

112 M.C. Shandala (reported by Dr Eldon Byrd) at the First International Symposium on the Biological Effects of Electromagnetic Radiation, Ottawa, June 1982.

113 Mizumori, S.J.Y., R. Lovely, R.B. Johnson and W. Guy, 'Developmental alterations in rats following in utero exposure to 500 µW/cm .2450 MHz microwaves', paper presented at the First Annual Meeting of the Bioelectromagnetic Society, Seattle, U.S.A., 18-22 June 1979.

114 Czerski, P.A., E. Manikowska-Gzerska and W.M. Leach, 'Effects of 0.915 and 0.4 GHz CW microwaves on meiosis in male mice', paper presented at the 5th Annual Meeting of the Bioelectromagnetic Society held in Boulder, Colorado, U.S.A., June 1983.

115 Lovely, T.H., R.B. Johnson, M. Mathews and W. Guy, 'Alteration of behavioural and biochemical parameters during and consequent to 500 µW/cm chronic 2450 MHz microwave exposure', paper presented at the International Symposium on Electromagnetic Waves and Biology, Ottawa, June 1978.

116 Dumansky, J.D. and M.G. Shandala, 'The biological action and hygienic significance of electromagnetic fields of super high and ultra high frequencies in densely populated areas', *Biologic Effects and Health Hazards of Microwave Radiation* (Warsaw, Polish Medical Publishers, 1974).

117 Guy, Arthur, in a paper presented at the Annual Meeting of the Bioelectromagnetic Society, Atlanta, Georgia, July 1984.

118 Szmigrelski, Stanislaw, et al, 'Accelerated development of spontaneous and benzopyrene-induced skin cancer in mice exposed to 2450 MHz microwave radiation', *Bioelectromagnetics*, 3.

119 Prausnitz, S. and C. Susskind, 'Effects of chronic microwave irradiation on mice', *IRE Transactions on Bio Medical Electronics*, 9.

120 Marha, J., J. Musil and H. Tuha, 'Electromagnetic fields and the life environment', *San Francisco Press* (1971).

121 Serdiuk, A.M., 'Biological effect of low-intensity ultrahigh frequency fields', *Crach Delo*, 11.

122 Lobanova, E.A. and A.V. Goncharova, 'Investigation of conditioned-reflex activity in animals (albino rats) subjected to the effect of ultrashort and short radio-waves', *Gig. Tr. Prof. Zabol*, 15, 1.

123 Demokidova, N.K., 'The effects of radiowaves on the growth of animals', in Z.V. Gordon (ed), *Biological Effects of Radiofrequency Electromagnetic Fields* (Arlington, Virginia, Joint Publications Research Service No. 63321).

124 Volkova, A.P. and P.O. Fukalova, 'Changes in certain protective reactions of an organism under the influence of MW in experimental and industrial conditions', in Z.V. Gordon, *Biological Effects of Radiofrequency Electromagnetic Fields* (Arlington, Virginia, Joint Publication Research Service No. 63321).

125 Durney, C.II., C.C. Johnson, et al, *Radiofrequency Radiation Dosimetry Handbook*, 2nd ed. (Brooks Air Force Base, School of Aerospace Medicine).

126 Marha, K., J. Musil and H. Tuha, *Electromagnetic Fields and the Life Environment* (Prague, State Health Publishing House).

127 Dietzel, F., W. Kern and R. Steckenmesser, 'Deformity and intrauterine death following short-wave therapy in early pregnancy in experimental animals', *Muench. Med Wochenschr.*, 114.

128 Varma, M.M. and E.A. Traboulay Jr., 'Biological effects of microwave radiation on the testes of Swiss mice', *Experientia*, 31 (1975).

129 National Radiological Protection Board, *Advice on the Protection of Workers and Members of the Public from the Possible Hazards of Electric and Magnetic Fields with Frequencies Below 300 GHz. A Consultative Document* (Chilton, 1986).

130 Michaelson, S.M., 'Health implications of exposure to radiowave and microwave energies', *British Journal of Industrial Medicine* (1982).

131 Cited in *Environmental Health Review*, 26, 1.

132 *Radiofrequency Sealers and Heaters. Potential Health Hazards and their Prevention.* Current Intelligence Bulletin 33. NIOSH/OSHA.

133 National Radiological Protection Board, *Advice on the Protection of Workers and Members of the Public from the Possible Hazards of Electric and Magnetic Fields with Frequencies Below 300 GHz.* (Chilton, 1986).

134 Czerski, P., 'Radiofrequency radiation exposure limits in Eastern Europe', *Journal of Microwave Power*, 20 (1985).

135 VDE 0848, Teil 2. (1984).

136 Reported by Dr Charles Graham, Kansas, U.S.A., Mid West Institute, 1990.

137 Reported by Dr Ross Adey, Professor of Medicine and White House Scientific Advisor on magnetic fields, Washington, 1990.

138 Reported by Dr Kjell Hansson-Mild, University of Umea, Sweden, 1989.

139 Guy, Arthur, W., *Health Hazards Assessment of Radio Frequency Electromagnetic Fields Emitted by Video Display Terminals* (Seattle, University of Washington).

140 Delgardo, J.M.R., J. Leal, J.L. Monteagudo and M.G. Gracia, 'Embryological changes induced by weak, extremely low frequency electromagnetic fields', *J. Anat.*, 134, (1983).

141 Juutilainen, J., M. Harris, K. Saali and T. Lahtinen, 'Effects of 100 Hz magnetic fields with various wave-forms on the development of chick embryos', *Radiat. Environ., and Biophysics*, 25 (1986).

142 Juutilainen, J. and K. Saali, 'Development of chick embryos in 1 Hz to 100 kHz magnetic fields', *Radiat. Environ., and Biophysics* (1986a).

143 Juutilainen, J. and K. Saali, 'Effects of low frequency magnetic fields on the development of chick embryos', in Knave and Wideback (eds), *op. cit.*

144 Mikolajnzk, H., J. Indulski, M. Pawlazyk and T. Kamedula, 'Effects of TV sets' electromagnetic fields on rats', in Knave and Wideback (eds), *op. cit.*

145 Mikolajnzk, H., J. Indulski, et al, 'Task-load and endocrinological risk for pregnancy in women VDU operators', in Knave and Wideback (eds), *op. cit.*

146 Milham, S., 'Mortality from leukaemia in workers related to electrical wires near homes', *International Journal of Epidemiology*, 11, 4.

147 Reported by Dr S. Milham, 1989.

148 Wright, W.E., J.M. Peterson and M. Mack Thomas, 'Leukaemia in workers exposed to electric and magnetic fields', *The Lancet*, 20 Nov. 1982.

149 Wertheimer, N. and E. Leeper, 'An increase in cancer rates among men in occupations with exposures to magnetic fields', *American Journal of Epidemiology* (1979).

150 Wertheimer, H. and E. Leeper, 'Adult cancer related to electrical wires near homes', *International Journal of Epidemiology*, 109, 4.

151 Wertheimer, H. and E. Leeper, 'Electrical wiring configurations and childhood cancer', *American Journal of Epidemiology*, 109, 4.

152 Adey, Ross, 'Frequency and power windowing in tissue interactions with weak electromagnetic fields', *Proceedings of IEEE 68* (1980).

153 Adey, Ross, 'Tissue interactions with non-ionizing electromagnetic fields', *Physiological Review*, 6, 2.

154 Adey, Ross, 'Molecular aspects of cell membranes as substances for interaction with electromagnetic fields', *Synergistic of the Brain* (Berlin, Springer).

155 Nordstrom, S., E. Birke and L. Gustavsson, 'Reproductive hazards among workers at high voltage substations', *Bioelectromagnetics* (1983).

156 R. Lin in a paper presented at the 1984 Annual Meeting of the Society for Risk Analysis, Knoxville, Tennesee, USA, reported in *Microwave News*, 4, 8.

157 Byrd, E., 'Review of the Soviet literature', in Proceedings of the International Forum on Low-level Radiation, Ottawa, June 1982.

158 Pearce (ed), *op. cit.*

159 Guy, Arthur, W., 'Health hazards of radio frequency electromagnetic fields emitted by video display terminals', in Knave and Wideback (eds), *op. cit.*

160 Ostberg, O., 'CRTs pose health problems for operators', *International Journal of Health and Safety*, Nov./Dec. 1975.

161 Zaret, M.M., 'Blindness, deafness and vestibular dysfunction in microwave workers', *The Eye, Ear, Nose and Throat Monthly*, 54 (1975).

162 Sadcikova, M.N., 'Clinical manifestations of reactions to microwave irradiation in various occupational groups', *Biological Effects and Health Hazards of Microwave Radiation* (Warsaw, Polish Medical Publishers, 1974).

163 Hirsch, F.G. and J.T. Parker, 'Bilateral lenticular opacities occurring in a technician operating a microwave generator', *Industrial Hygiene*, 6 (1952).

164 Carpenter, R.L. and D.D. Donaldson, 'Bilateral cataracts following microwave diathermy treatments: a case history', paper presented at the 5th International Symposium, Scheveningen, The Netherlands, of the International Microwave Power Institute.

165 Zaret, M.M., 'Selected cases of microwave cataract in man associated with concomitant annotated pathologies', in *Biological Effects and Health Hazards of Microwave Radiation* (1974).

166 Duke-Elder, S., 'The pathological action (of radiant energy) upon the lens', *The Lancet*, 1 (1926).

167 Bouchat, J. and C. Marsol, '9199670: Cataracts capsulair bilaterale et radar', *Archives d'Opthalmologue de Paris*, 27.

168 Zaret, M.M., 'Cataracts and visual display units', in Pearce (ed), *op. cit.*

169 'EEC Council Directive on the minimum safety and health requirements for work with display screen equipment (Fifth Individual Directive within the meaning of Article 16 (1) of Directive 87/391/EEC) 90/270/EEC', *Official Journal of the European Communities*, L.156/14, 29 May 1990.

170 Lee, W.R., 'Working with display units', *British Medical Journal*, 12 Oct. 1985.

171 Saunders, R.D. and M. Smith, 'Safety aspects of NMR clinical imaging', *British Medical Bulletin*, 40 (1984).

172 Bompard, Paul, 'US adits radiation build-up at air bases', *The Times*, 18 July 1988.

173 Smith, Iola, 'Tiling over the deadly gas cracks', *The Times*, 6 Dec. 1990.

174 Tytler, D., 'Radon alert', *The Times*, 3 Dec. 1990.

175 United Kingdom Atomic Energy Authority, *The Effects and Control of Radiation*, 2nd ed. (The Southern Publishing Co., Westminster Press, 1986).

176 Coghill, R., *Electropollution* (Thorsons Publishers, 1990).

177 Hawkins, L.H., 'The influence of air ions, temperature, and humidity on selective well being and comfort', *Jnl. Environ. Psychology* (1981).

178 Hawkins, L.H., 'The possible benefit of negative-ion generators', in Pearce (ed), *op. cit.*

179 United Kingdom Atomic Energy Authority, *Radiation and Medicine* (London, U.K.A.E.A., 1991).

180 J. Shelmerdine, Radiological Protection Service, Manchester University, in conversations with the author during 1990/91.

181 McKie, Robin, 'Britain's deadly Chernobyl legacy', *Sunday Observer*, 21 April 1991.

182 Hawkes, Nigel, 'Radon gas hot spots found', *The Times*, 19 May 1991.

183 Savitz, D., 'Leukaemia and occupational exposure to electromagnetic fields; review of epidemiological surveys', *Journal of Occupational Medicine*, 29, 1 (1987).

184 Savitz, D., 'Childhood cancer and electromagnetic field exposure', *Journal of Epidemiology* (1988).

185 Huws, Ursula, *VDU Hazards Handbook* (London Hazards Centre Trust, 1987).

186 Marha, K., J. Musil and H. Tuha, *Electromagnetic Fields and the Life Environment* (San Francisco Press, 1971).

187 Thomas, Burch and Yeandle, 'Microwave radiation and chlordiazepoxide: synergistic effects on fixed-internal behaviour', *Science* (1979).

188 Mangold, Tom, 'Electricity: A shock in store', *B.B.C. T.V. Panorama Programme*, 21 March 1988.

189 Smith, Iola, 'Stripping down a radiation risk', *The Sunday Times*, 6 Nov. 1988.

190 Nuttall, Nick, 'Electrical gremlins drive machines mad', *The Times*, 9 July 1991.

191 *Handbook* (London, Electricity Council, 1988).

Part Four

Chapter 19: There's going to be a revolution

1 'EEC Council Directive on the minimum safety and health requirements for work with display screen equipment (Fifth Individual Directive within the meaning of Article 16 (1) of Directive 87/391/EEC) 90/270/EEC', *Official Journal of the European Communities*, L.156/14, 29 May 1990.

2 Turiel, I., C.G. Hollowell, et al, 'The effects of reduced ventilation on indoor air quality in an office building', *Atmospheric Environment*, 17.

3 Grandjean, E. and E. Vigliani (eds), *Ergonomics and Health in Modern Offices* (London, Taylor and Francis, 1984).

4 Ishai, E., 'The effects of VDU on the interior design of offices', in Knave and Wideback (eds), *op. cit.*

5 Pendreigh, B., 'Computer faults could kill', *The Scotsman*, 13 June 19909.

6 DeMatteo, *op. cit.*

7 The Orbit Report, *Planning the Office of the Future Today* (London, Steelcase Strafor, 1990).

8 Waters, C.R., 'Just when you thought it was safe to go back to the office', *INC Magazine*, Jan. 1983.

9 *Working with Display Units*, Occupational Safety and Health Series No. 61 (Geneva, International Labour Office, 1989).

10 *Bundesgesetzblatt*, 354 (1981).

11 'Amélioration des conditions de travail sur les postes du type terminal-écran' (France, Institut National de Recherche Scientifique).

12 *VDUs at Work*, Occupational Safety and Health Working Environment Series 13 (Australia, Dept. of Employment and Industrial Relations, 1983).

13 *VDT Work and Occupational Health* (Japan, Labour Ministry Central Council of Labour Standards, 1984).

14 'In the chips: opportunities, people partnerships', *Microelectronics and Employment* (Canada, Labour Canada Task Force, 1982).

15 *Recommendations Concerning Work with VDUs* (Canadian Centre for Occupational Health and Safety, 1983).

16 *Guide d'aménagement de postes de travail à écran cathodique* (Commission de Santé et de la Securité du Québec, 1982).

17 Duane, T.D. and T. Behrendt, 'Extrasensory electroencephalographic induction between identical twins', *Science*, Oct. 1965.

18 Dr Wilfreid Kreisel, World Federation of Building Contractors, at a meeting in Birmingham, June 1990.

19 Bertell, Rosalie, 'The health hazards of video display terminals', *Environmental Health Review*, 26, 1 (1982).

Chapter 20: Essential subsidiary equipment

1 'EEC Council Directive on the minimum safety and health requirements for work with display screen equipment (Fifth Individual Directive within the meaning of Article 16 (1) of Directive 87/391/EEC) 90/270/EEC', *Official Journal of the European Communities*, L.156/14, 29 May 1990.

2 The Orbit Report, *Planning the Office of the Future Today* (London, Steelcase Strafor, 1990).

3 Waters, C.R., 'Just when you thought it was safe to go back in the office' *INC Magazine*, Jan. 1983.
4 *Working with Visual Display Units*, Occupational Safety and Health Series No. 61 (Geneva, International Labour Office, 1989).
5 Wahlberg, J.E. and C. Linden, 'VDU work and the skin', in Knave and Wideback (eds), *op. cit.*

Chapter 22: The chair, the desk and power at your fingertips

1 *Meubles de Bureau*, CEN., EN 91 (Paris, La Defence, 1981).
2 Dreyfuss, H., *Designing for People* (New York, Simon and Schuster).
3 Snorrason, E., 'Hvilestolsproblemer', *Tidsskrift for Danske Sygehuse* (1968).
4 Mandal, A.C., 'What is the correct height of furnit9ure?', in E. Grandjean and E. Vigliani (eds), *Ergonomics and Health in Modern Offices* (London, Taylor and Francis, 1984).
5 Hansson, T., 'The back during prolonged sitting', in Knave and Wideback (eds), *op. cit.*
6 Middleton, Scott, British Chiropractic Association, to the author, Nov. 1990.
7 Ishai, E., 'The effect of the VDU on the interior design of offices', in Knave and Wideback (eds), *op. cit.*
8 Bridger, R.S., D. Wilkinson and T. Van Houweninge, 'Hip joint mobility and spinal angles in standing and in different sitting postures', *Human Factors*, 31, 2 (1989).
9 Adams, M.A. and W.C. Hutton, 'The effect of posture on the lumbar spine', *Journal of Bone and Joint Surgery*, 67B (1985).
10 Grandjean, E., W. Hunting and M. Piedermann, 'VDT workstation design: preferred settings and their effects', *Human Factors*, 25 (1983).
11 Dainoff, M.J. and M.A. Leonard, 'Task and the adjustment of ergonomic chairs', in Knave and Wideback (eds), *op. cit.*
12 *Working with Display Units*, Occupational Safety and Health Series No. 61 (Geneva, International Labour Office, 1989).
13 'EEC Council Directive on the minimum safety and health requirements for work with display screen equipment (Fifth Individual Directive within the meaning of Article 16 (1) of Directive 87/391/EEC) 90/270/EEC', *Official Journal of the European Communities*, L.156/14, 29 May 1990.
14 Mandal, A.C., 'What is the correct height of furniture?', in E. Grandjean and E. Vigliani (eds), *Ergonomics and Health in Modern Offices* (London, Taylor and Francis, 1984).
15 Cakir, A., et al, *Visual Display Terminals* (London, John Wiley).
16 *Meubles de Bureau*, Paris, France. La Defence. C.E.N. EN91. 1981.
17 Dreyfuss, H., *Designing for People* (New York, Simon and Schuster).
18 Snorrason, E., 'Hvilestolsproblemer', *Tidsskrift for Danske Sygehuse* (1968).
19 Gordon Russell plc, Broadway, Worcestershire WR12 7AD. Telephone 0386-858483.
20 Steelcase Strafor (UK) Ltd., 100 Avenue Road, Swiss Cottage, London NW3 3HF. Telephone 081-586 5933.

Chapter 24: Noise

1 *Code of Practice for Reducing the Exposure of Employed Persons to Noise* (London, Health and Safety Executive, 1972, rep. 1978).

2 *Working with Visual Display Units*, Occupational Safety and Health Series No. 61 (Geneva, International Labour Office, 1989).

3 *Health and Safety for White Collar Workers*, FIET Handbook No. 1 (Geneva, International Federation of Commercial, Clerical, Professional and Technical Employees, 1983).

4 Gasaway, D.C., 'Noise induced hearing loss', in Robert J. McCunney (ed), *Handbook of Occupational Medicine* (Boston/Toronto, Little, Brown and Co., 1988).

5 Gasaway, D.C., *Hearing Conversation: A Practical Manual and Guide* (Englewood Cliffs, N.J., Prentice-Hall, 1985).

6 Alberti, P.W., 'Noise and the ear', in J. Ballantyne and Groves (eds), *Scott-Brown's Diseases of the Ear, Nose and Throat*, 4th ed. (Boston, Butterworth, 1979). Vol. 2, pp 551-622.

7 Cohen, A., J. Anticaglia and E.E. Jones, 'Sociocusis: hearing loss from non-occupational noise exposure', *Sound Vibration*, 4, 11 (1970).

8 American Academy of Otolaryngology – Head and Neck Surgery Foundation Inc., *Guide for Conservation of Hearing in Noise*, rev. ed. (Rochester, Maine, Custom Printing, 1982). With Addendum, 1983.

9 Silverman, S.R., 'Rehabilitative audiology', in M.M. Paparella and Shumrick (eds), *Otolaryngology*, 2nd ed. (Philadelphia, Saunders, 1980).

10 'Noise pollution: irritant or hazard?', *Harvard Medical School Health Letter*, 11, 8 (1986).

11 *Noise: Environmental Health Criteria*, 12 (Geneva, World Health Organization, 1980).

12 *Occupational Noise Exposure: Hearing Conservation Amendment; Final Rule. Fed. Reg. 48(946):9737-85*, 8 March 1983.

13 *Guides to the Evaluation of Permanent Impairment*, 2nd ed. (Chicago, American Medical Association, 1984).

14 *Criteria for Recommended Standard-Occupational Exposure to Noise* (Washington, D.C., National Institute of Occupational Safety and Health, 1972).

15 DeMatteo, *op. cit.*

16 'The ultrasound risk', *Microwave News*, 4, 2 (1984).

17 Liebeskind, D., et al, 'Sister chromatid exchange in human lymphocytes after exposure to diagnostic ultrasound', *Science*, 205 (1979).

18 Ciaravino, V., et al, 'Diagnostic ultrasound and sister chromatid exchanges: failure to reproduce positive findings', *Science*, 227 (1985).

19 Gasaway, Donald C., 'Noise-induced hearing loss', in Robert J. McCunney (ed), *Handbook of Occupational Medicine* (Boston/Toronto, Little, Brown and Co., 1988).

Chapter 25: Lighting

1 Swedish National Board for Occupational Safety and Health, *Reading of Display Screens*, Directive 136.

2 *Guidance Notes: Visual Display Screens* (London, Health and Safety Executive, 1983).

3 London and Home Counties Area Technology Sub-Committee, Association of Professional, Executive, Clerical and Computer Staff, *New Technology: A Health and Safety Report* (1985).

4 Bjorset, Hans-Henrik, 'Lighting for visual display unit workplaces', in Knave and Wideback (eds), *op. cit.*

5 Boyce, Peter, R., *Lighting the display or displaying the lighting* (Chester, Electricity Council Research Centre).

6 Van Ooyen, M.H.F. and S.H.A. Bergemann, *Lighting the electronic office* (Eindhoven, Philips International).

7 Bergemann, S.H.A. and R.T. A. Hendriks, 'The ups and downs of office lighting', in *Proceedings of the National Lighting Conference 1984* (London, The Chameleon Press, 1984).

8 Hedge, A., 'Office health hazards', *Ergonomics*, 30, 4 (1987).

9 Kuller, Rikard, *Non visual effects of visual surroundings* (Lund Institute of Technology, 1986).

10 Gerard, R.M., 'Differential effects of coloured lights on psychophysiological functions', University of California Los Angeles doctoral dissertation.

11 Ali, M.R., 'Pattern of EEG recovery under photic stimulation by light of different colours', *Electroencheph. Clin. Neurophysiol*, 33.

12 Lacey, J.I., et al, 'The visceral level: situational determinant and behavioural correlates of autonomic response patterns', in P.H. Knapp (ed), *Expression of the Emotions in Man* (New York, International Universities Press).

13 Hollwich, F., *The influence of ocular light perception on metabolism in man and in animal* (Berlin, Springer-Verlag).

14 Wurtman, R.J., 'The effect of light on the human body', *Scientific American*, 233, 1.

15 Kuller, R., 'Non visual effects of light and colour', Document D.15 (Stockholm, Swedish Council for Building Research).

16 Wetterberg, L., 'Melatonin in humans, Physiological clinical studies', *Journal of Neural Transmission*, suppl. 13.

17 Hollwich, F., B. Dieckhues and B. Schrameyer, 'Die Würkung des natürlichen und kunstlichen Lichtes über das Auge auf den Hormon – und Stoffwechselhaushalt des Menschen', *Klin. Mbl Augenheilkunde*, 171.

18 Stone, P.T., et al, 'Light, endocrine mechanisms and stress', *Report No. 156* (Loughborough University).

19 Sugimoto, S. and I. Ikeda, 'Illuminance and physiological load', *Proc. CIE 20th Session*, Vol. 1, D602, 1-4.

20 Erikson, C. and R. Kuller, 'Non visual effects of office lighting', *Proc. CIE 20th Session*, Vol. 2, D602, 1-4.

21 Kuller, R., 'Hur inverkar belysningen pa manniskan? Miljopsykologisk forskning vid Sektion', *A. Ordo*, 2.

22 Lindsten, C. and R. Kuller, *Health impact on schoolchildren from lack of natural daylight* (Lund Institute of Technology).

23 Brundett, G.W., 'Human sensitivity to flicker', *Lighting Research and Technology*, 6, 3.

24 United States Department of Health and Human Services, *Potential Health Hazards of Video Display Terminals*, Publication No. 81-129 (Cincinnati, National Institute for Occupational Safety and Health, 1981).

25 'Special issue on visual display units', *Conditions of Work Digest*, 5, 1 (Geneva, International Labour Office, 1986).

26 Gunnarson, E. and O. Ostberg, *The Physical and Psychological Working Environment in a Terminal-Based Computer Storage and Retrieval System*, Report 35 (Stockholm, National Board of Occupational Safety and Health, 1977).

27 Cakir, A., et al, *The VDT Manual* (Darmstadt, Ince-Fiej Research Association, 1979).

28 Laubli, T., 'Visual impairments related to environmental conditions in VDU operators', in E. Grandjean and E. Vigliani (eds), *Ergonomic Aspects of Visual Display Terminals* (London, Taylor and Francis, 1980).

29 Elias, R., et al, 'Conditions de travail devant les écrans cathodiques: organisation des taches et astreintes de l'organisme', *Cahiers de Notes Documentaires*, 101 (1980).

30 Stammerjohn, L.W., M.J. Smith and B.G.F. Cohen, 'Evaluation of workstation design factors in VDT operations', *Humane Factors*, we, 4 (1981).

31 Ostberg, O., 'Fatigue in clerical work in CRT display terminals', *Göteborg Psychological Report*, 4, 19 (1974).

32 Godefroy, M., 'Ecrans et ergonomie, un effet de coherence et deharmonisation virant l'amelioration des postes de travail', *Travail et Securité*, 7/8 (1984).

33 Mayer, J.J., et al, 'L'analyse ergonomique des postes de travail avec l'écran de visualisation', *Cahiers Ecotra*, Publication IMSP No. 214 (1980).

34 United States Military Standard, *Human Engineering Design Criteria for Military Systems and Equipment* (Washington, D.C., United States Department of Defense).

35 *Working with Visual Display Units*, Occupational Safety and Health Series No. 61 (Geneva, International Labour Office, 1989).

Chapter 26: The sick building syndrome

1 'EEC Council Directive on the minimum safety and health requirements for work with display screen equipment (Fifth Individual Directive within the meaning of Article 16 (1) of Directive 87/391/EEC) 90/270/EEC', *Official Journal of the European Communities*, L.156/14, 29 May 1990.

2 Turiel, I., C.G. Hollowell, et al, 'The effects of reduced ventilation on indoor air quality in an office building', *Atmospheric Environment*, 17.

3 Mandal, A.C., 'What is the correct height of furniture?', in E. Grandjean and E. Vigliani (eds), *Ergonomics and Health in Modern Offices* (London, Taylor and Francis, 1984).

4 Ishai, E., 'The effects of VDU on the interior design of offices', in Knave and Wideback (eds), *op. cit.*

5 Pendreigh, B., 'Computer faults could kill', *The Scotsman*, 13 June 1990.

6 DeMatteo, *op. cit.*

7 Rufford, N., 'Legion bug could be wiped out by £30 test', *Sunday Times*, 22 May 1988.

8 Wilson, S., *Office Environment Study* (London, Building Use Studies).

9 Wilson, S., *Premises of Excellence* (London, Building Use Studies).

10 Schneider, T., 'Manmade mineral fibre and other fibers in the air and in settled dust', *Environment International* (1988). Papers presented at the International Conference on Indoor Air quality and Climate, Stockholm, Sweden, published by Pergamon Journals, Virginia, U.S.A.

11 Laforce, F. Marc, 'Airborne infections and modern building technology', *Environment International* (1988).

12 Berglund, B. and T. Lindvall, 'Sensory reactions to sick buildings', *Environment International* (1988).

13 Molhave, L., B. Bach and O.F. Pedersen, 'Human reactions to low concentration of volatile organic compounds', *Environment International* (1988).

14 Berg-Munch, B., G. Clausen and P.O. Fanger, 'Ventilation requirements for the control of body odour in spaces occupied by women', *Environment International* (1988).

15 Goldstein, I.F., D. Hartel, L.R. Andrews and A.L. Weinstein, 'Indoor air pollution exposures of low-income inner-city residents', *Environment International* (1988).

16 Flachsbart, P.G. and R.O. Wayne, 'A rapid method for surveying CO concentration in high-rise buildings', *Environment International* (1988).

17 Meyer, B., 'Formaldehyde exposure from building products', *Environment International* (1988).

18 Levin, H. and J. Hahn, 'Pentachlorophenol in indoor air. Methods to reduce airborne concentrations', *Environment International* (1988).

19 Fugas, M., 'Assessment of true human exposure to air pollution', *Environment International* (1988).

20 Skaaret, E., 'Contaminant removal performance in terms of ventilation effectiveness', *Environment International* (1988).

21 Hedge, A. in *Ergonomics*, 30, 5 (1987).

22 Hedge, A., 'Office design: user reactions to open plan', in R. Thorne and S. Aden (eds), *People and the ManMade Environment. Building Urban and Landscape Design related to Human Behaviour* (University of Sydney).

23 Hedge, A., 'The impact of design on employee reactions to their offices', in J. Winerman (ed), *Behaviour Issues in Office Design* (New York, Van Nostrand-Rhinehold).

24 Hedge, A., 'A systematic investigation of employee reactions to their work environment', *Environment and Behaviour*, 14.

25 A. Hedge, reported in *Ergonomics*, 30, 5.

26 Tomlinson, M., 'Critical conditions', summary of a BBC 2 investigation into sick building syndrome, *The Listener*, 27 April 1989.

27 Gunn, S., 'Call for radon enquiry', *The Times*, 20 June 1990.

28 Hurrell, M., 'Does your work make you sick', *The Times*, 14 June 1990.

29 Shrimsley, R., 'Trend for air conditioning helps spread deadly bug', *Sunday Telegraph*, 3 March 1989.

30 Baker, B., 'Case history: I love my work – it's just the office I hate', *Best Magazine*, 2 Feb. 1990.

31 Orbit Research Document, *Planning the Office of the Future Today* (London, Orbit Research Group, 1990).

32 Hatch, T.F. and P. Gross, *Pulmonary Deposition and Retention of Aerosols* (New York, Academic 1964).

33 Brockton, L., D. Weisenberger and C. Gray, 'The establishment of an occupational health program', *Hand-book of Occupational Medicine* (Boston/Toronto, Little, Brown and Co., 1988).

34 *Les Ecrans de Visualisation, Guide Méthodologique pour le Médicin du Travail* (Paris, Institut National de Recherche et de Sécurité, 1984).

35 *Working with Visual Display Units*, Occupational Safety and Health Series No. 61 (Geneva, International Labour Office, 1989).

36 Godefroy, M., 'Ecrans et ergonomie, un effet de cohérence et déharmonisation virant l'amélioration des postes de travail', *Travail et Sécurité* (1984).

37 International Federation of Commercial, Clerical, Professional and Technical Employees (FIET) International Trade Union Conference paper on visual display units, Geneva, 1984.

38 Coghill, R., *Electropollution* (London, Thorsons Publishers, 1990).

39 Brock, G., 'Death sentence for the Brussels Berlaymonster', *The Times*, 30 April 1991.

40 Matthews, Robert,, 'Legionella link to building-site dust', *The Times*, 1 July 1988.

41 Oldfield, Stephen, 'Killer disease fear closes jet factory', *Daily Mail*, 6 Oct. 1988.

42 Smith, Ian, 'Legionnaires fear shuts BAe plant', *The Times*, 6 Oct. 1988.

43 McKee, Victoria, 'Sickness in the bricks', *The Times*, 11 Aug. 1988.

Index

(1) General

(2) Medical problems